The Ultimate Anti-inflammatory Diet Cookbook

East and Complete anti-inflammatory meal plan to reset metabolism, lose weight fast and regain confidence in a few steps

Polly Arnold

© Copyright 2021 - All rights reserved

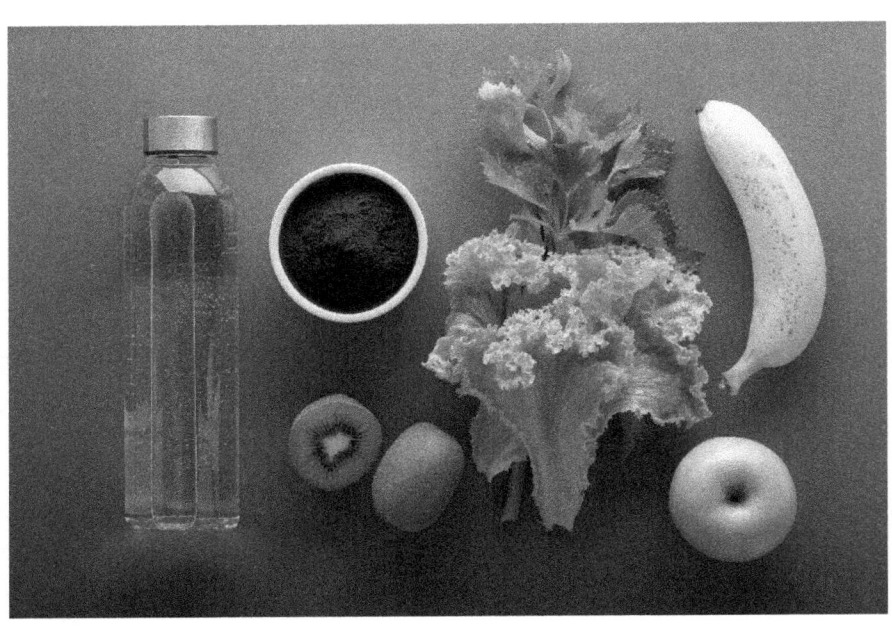

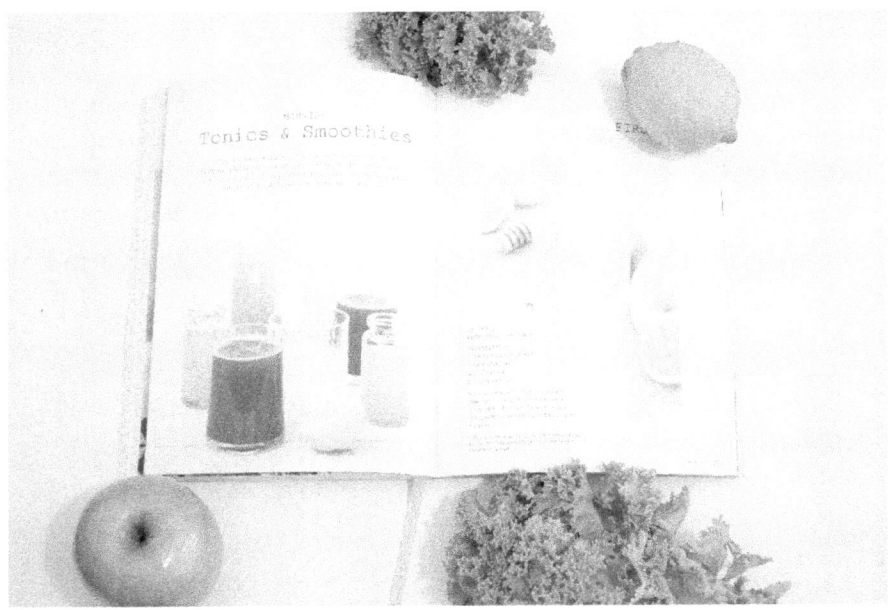

Table Of Contents

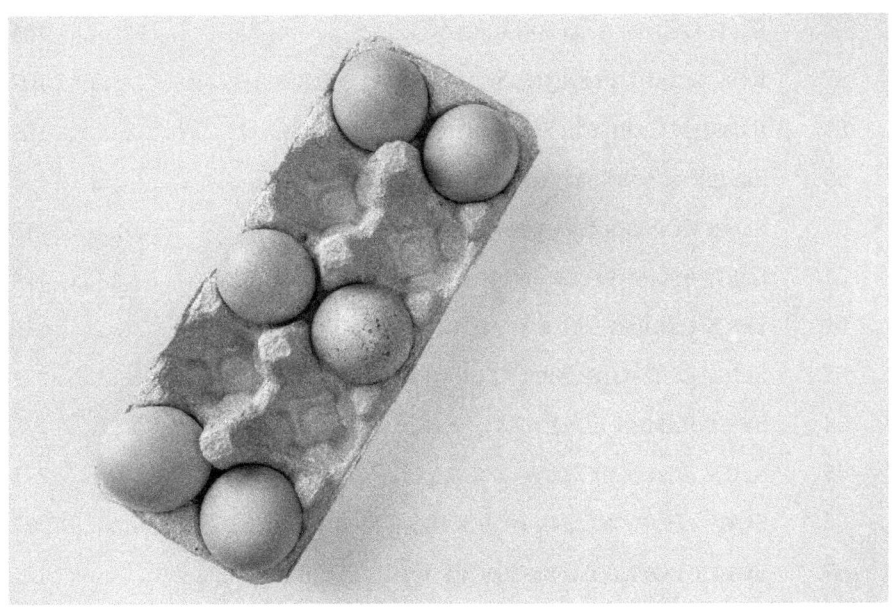

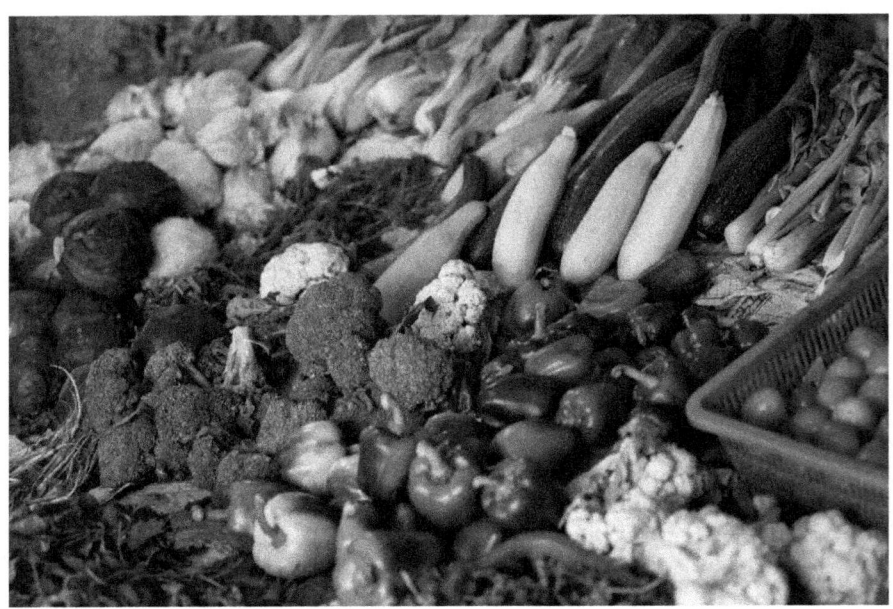

<u>Recipes</u>

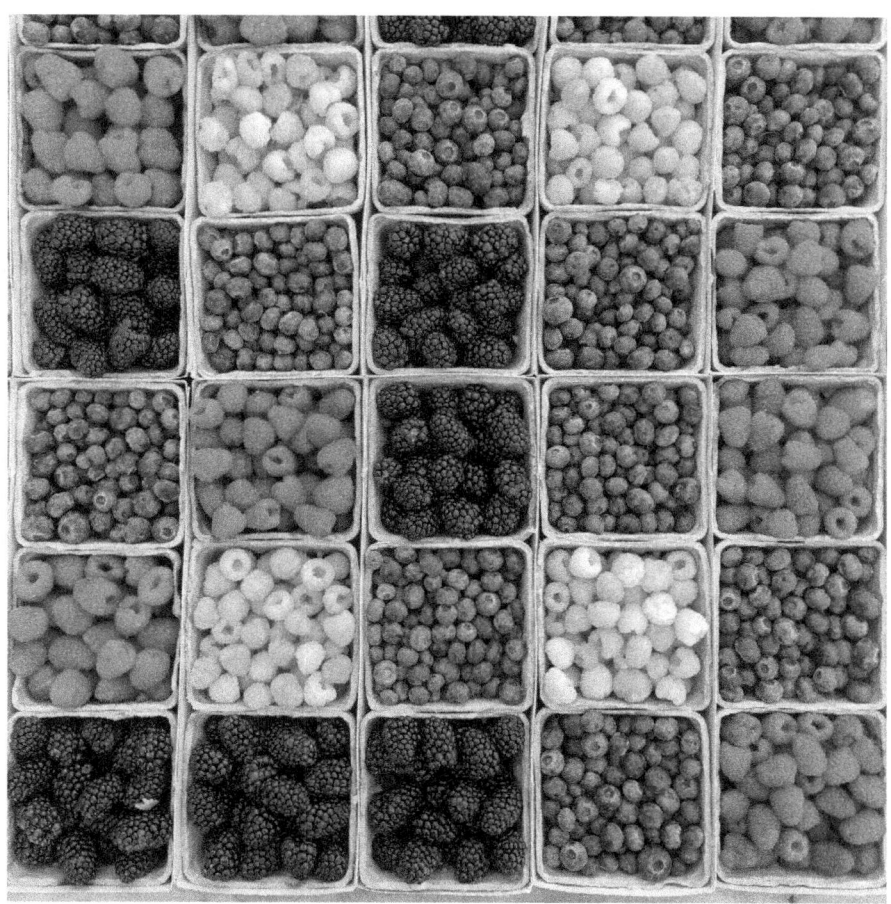

1. CHEESY BROCCOLI SOUP

Time To Prepare: five minutes

Time to Cook: twenty minutes **Yield:** Servings 4

Ingredients:

- 1 cup broccoli, cut into florets

- 1 cup chicken broth

- 1 cup heavy whipping cream

- 1 cup shredded Cheddar cheese, plus more for topping • 2 tablespoons butter

- From the cupboard:

- Salt and freshly ground black pepper, to taste

Directions:

1. Place the butter in a deep cooking pan, and melt on moderate heat.

2. Put in and sauté the broccoli for four to five minutes or until tender.

3. Stir in the chicken broth and heavy whipping cream over the broccoli, and drizzle with salt and black pepper. Cook for approximately fifteen minutes or until the soup is smooth and thickened. Keep stirring during the cooking.

4. Lower the heat to low and gently fold in the Cheddar cheese. Keep stirring until well blended.

5. Ladle the soup into a big container. Spread more cheese over the soup before you serve.

Nutritional Info: calories: 386 , total fat: 37.3g , total carbs: 3.8g , fiber: 1.1g , net carbs: 2.7g , protein: 9.8g

2. CHEESY CHICKEN SOUP

Time To Prepare: twenty minutes

Time to Cook: 33-40 minutes **Yield:** Servings 6

Ingredients:

- ¼ teaspoon black pepper

- ½ cup shredded cheddar cheese

- ½ teaspoon cumin

- ½ teaspoon salt

- 1 cup whipped cream cheese

- 1 tablespoon coconut oil, for cooking

- 1 teaspoon chili powder

- 1 yellow onion, chopped

- 2 boneless, skinless chicken breasts

- 2 cloves garlic, chopped

- 2 cups chicken broth

- 2 cups water

Directions:

1. Heat a big frying pan on moderate heat with a ½ tablespoon of the coconut oil.

2. Brown the chicken breasts until thoroughly cooked. Set aside.

3. Put in the garlic and onion to a big stockpot with the rest of the 1 tablespoon of the coconut oil and sauté until translucent over low to moderate heat. This should take about three to five minutes.

4. Put in this chicken broth and water.

5. Whisk in the cream cheese and keep whisking over low to moderate heat until blended.

6. Put in in the spices and bring to its boiling point.

7. While the water is boiling, chop the chicken into bite-sized pieces and put in to the stockpot.

8. Reduce to a simmer and cook for half an hour.

9. Mix in the cheddar cheese before you serve.

Nutritional Info: Calories: 157 , Carbohydrates: 5g , Fiber: 1g Net , Carbohydrates: 4g , Fat: 7g , Protein: 17g

3. CHEESY TOMATO AND BASIL SOUP

Time To Prepare: five minutes

Time to Cook: fifteen minutes **Yield:** Servings 12

Ingredients:

- ¼ teaspoon ground black pepper

- 1 tablespoon dried basil

- 1 teaspoon dried oregano

- 1 teaspoon salt

- 2 (14 ounces / 397 g) canned whole tomatoes, diced

- 2 garlic cloves, minced

- 2 tablespoons coconut oil

- 4 cups chicken broth

- 4 ounces (113 g) red onions, finely diced

- 5 ounces (142 g) grated Parmesan cheese, plus more for decoration

- 8 ounces (227 g) cream cheese, softened

- Fresh basil, chopped, for decoration

Directions:

1. Grease a nonstick frying pan with coconut oil, and sauté the onions, basil, oregano, and garlic in the frying pan for about four minutes or until aromatic. 2. Put in the cream cheese and fully whisk until no clump,

then fold in the chicken broth, and put in the cheese, tomatoes, salt, and pepper. Stir to blend well.

3. Cover the lid and bring them to a simmer on moderate heat for eight minutes. Move the soup into a blender, then blitz until it becomes thick.

4. Lightly pour the soup into a big serving container and sprinkle with Parmesan cheese and basil as decorate.

Nutritional Info: calories: 146 , total fat: 12g , net carbs: 3g , fiber: 1g , protein: 6g

4. CHICKEN AND CAULIFLOWER CURRY STEW

Time To Prepare: fifteen minutes

Time to Cook: 4 hours **Yield:** Servings 7

Ingredients:

- ¼ cup fresh cilantro, chopped

- ⅓ cup coconut oil

- 1 green bell pepper, chopped

- 1 pound (454 g) cauliflower, chopped into little pieces

- 1.5pounds (680 g) skinless, boneless chicken thighs, cut into bite-sized pieces

- 14 ounces (397 g) unsweetened coconut milk

- 2 tablespoons curry powder

- 2 tablespoons ginger garlic paste • Salt and ground black pepper, to taste

Directions:

1.   Warm half of the coconut oil in a nonstick frying pan on moderate heat, then sauté the garlic ginger paste and curry powder for a minutes or until aromatic.

2.   Put in the chicken pieces, and drizzle with salt and pepper. sauté for another ten minutes or until the chicken is mildly browned. Remove from the frying pan and set aside in warm.

3.   Warm another half of coconut oil in the frying pan, then sauté the cauliflower and bell pepper on moderate to high heat for one to two minutes. 4. Then fold in the coconut milk and reduce the heat to low. Cover with lid and stew for about fortyfive minutes.

5. Drizzle with salt and pepper, then put in the sautéed chicken. Move the stew to a big platter and serve with cilantro on top as decorate.

Nutritional Info: calories: 782 , total fat: 68g , net carbs: 9g , fiber: 5g , protein: 33g

5. CHICKEN AND KALE SOUP

Time To Prepare: five minutes

Time to Cook: 4 hours **Yield:** Servings 4

Ingredients:

- 1 (7-ounce / 198-g) bunch kale, trimmed and chopped

- 1 big chicken breast, cut into little strips

- 2 tablespoons olive oil

- 3 tablespoons fresh ginger, grated

- 6 cups chicken stock

- 6 garlic cloves, finely chopped

- From the cupboard:

- Salt and freshly ground black pepper, to taste

Directions:

1. Grease the insert of the slow cooker with olive oil.

2. Combine the chicken breast, stock, kale, ginger, garlic, ginger, salt, and black pepper in the slow cooker.

3. Place the slow cooker lid on and cook on HIGH for 4 hours.

4. Ladle the stew in a big container and serve warm.

Nutritional Info: calories: 168 , total fat: 7.6g , total carbs: 8.3g , fiber: 2.1g , net carbs: 6.2g , protein: 18.7g

6. CHICKEN CHILI BLANCO

Time To Prepare: ten minutes **Time to Cook:** twenty minutes **Yield:** Servings 4

Ingredients:

- ¼ teaspoon cayenne pepper

- 1 tablespoon ghee

- 1 teaspoon chili powder

- 2 (4-ounce) cans diced mild green chiles with their liquid

- 2 scallions, cut

- 2 small onions, chopped

- 2 teaspoons dried oregano

- 4 cups chicken broth or vegetable broth

- 4 cups shredded cooked chicken

- 4 cups white beans, drained and washed well

- 4 teaspoons ground cumin

- 6 garlic cloves, minced

Directions:

1. In a huge soup pot on moderate heat, melt the ghee.

2. Put in the onions and garlic, and sauté for five minutes.

3. Place the chiles, and cook for a couple of minutes, stirring.

4. Mix in the beans, broth, cumin, oregano, chili powder, and cayenne pepper. Heat it until it simmers.

5. Put in the chicken, bring to a simmer, decrease the heat to moderate-low, and cook for about ten minutes. Serve instantly, sprinkled with the scallions.

Nutritional Info: Calories: 304 , Total Fat: 4g , Saturated Fat: 2g , Cholesterol: 0mg , Carbohydrates: 46g , Fiber: 12g , Protein: 21g

7. CHICKEN TORTILLA SOUP

Time To Prepare: ten minutes **Time to Cook:** twenty minutes **Yield:** Servings 8-10

Ingredients:

- 1 teaspoon cayenne pepper or to taste

- 2 cups onions, chopped

- 2 teaspoons chili powder

- 2 teaspoons cumin powder

- 2 teaspoons dried oregano

- 2 teaspoons garlic powder

- 4 cups carrots, cut

- 4 cups celery, cut

- 4 cups water

- 4 teaspoons olive oil

- 6 cups rotisserie chicken, skinless, chopped or shredded

- 8 cloves garlic, minced

- 8 cups chicken broth

- 8 medium tomatoes, chopped

- Avocado, peeled, pitted, chopped

- For the topping: Use any (not necessary)

- Fresh cilantro, chopped

- Greek yogurt

- Pepper powder to taste

- Salt to taste

- Tortilla chips, crumbled

Directions:

1. Put a soup pot on moderate heat. Put in oil.

2. When the oil is warmed, put the onion and celery and sauté until slightly soft.

3. Put in garlic and sauté for a few seconds until aromatic. Stir in the tomatoes and cook until tender. Remove the heat.

4. Move into a blender. Put in water and blend until the desired smoothness is achieved.

5. Put back the mixed mixture into the pot. Put in the remaining ingredients and stir.

6. If it's beginning to boil, reduce the heat then simmer until vegetables are tender.

7. Ladle into soup bowls before you serve.

Nutritional Info: Calories: 1593 kcal , Protein: 147.22 g , Fat: 102.27 g , Carbohydrates: 13.17 g

8. CHICKPEA CURRY SOUP

Time To Prepare: ten minutes

Time to Cook: twenty-five minutes **Yield:** Servings 4

Ingredients:

- ¼ cup extra-virgin olive oil or coconut oil

- 1 (fifteen-ounce) can chickpeas, drained and washed

- 1 big apple, cored, peeled, and slice into ¼-inch dice

- 1 cup full-fat coconut milk

- 1 medium onion, finely chopped

- 1 teaspoon salt

- 2 garlic cloves, cut

- 2 tablespoons finely chopped fresh cilantro

- 2 teaspoons curry powder

- 3 cups peeled butternut squash cut into ½-inch dice

- 3 cups vegetable broth

Directions:

1. In a large pot, heat the oil on high heat.

2. Put in the onion and garlic and sauté until the onion starts to brown, six to eight minutes.

3. Place the apple, curry powder, and salt and sauté to toast the curry powder, one to two minutes.

4. Place the squash and broth then bring to its boiling point.

5. Reduce the heat then cook until the squash is soft about ten minutes.

6. Mix in the coconut milk.

7. Use an immersion blender to purée the soup in the pot until the desired smoothness is achieved.

8. Mix in the chickpeas and cilantro, heat through for one to two minutes, before you serve.

Nutritional Info: Calories: 469 , Total Fat: 30g , Total Carbohydrates: 45g , Sugar: 14g , Fiber: 10g , Protein: 12g , Sodium: 1174mg

9. CLEAR CLAM CHOWDER

Time To Prepare: ten minutes

Time to Cook: fifteen minutes **Yield:** Servings 4

Ingredients:

- ¼ teaspoon freshly ground black pepper

- ½ teaspoon dried thyme

- ½ teaspoon salt

- 1 (10-ounce) can clams

- 1 (8-ounce) bottle clam juice

- 1 small red onion, cut into ¼-inch dice

- 2 celery stalks, thinly cut

- 2 cups vegetable broth

- 2 garlic cloves, cut

- 2 medium carrots, cut into ½-inch pieces

- 2 tablespoons unsalted butter

Directions:

1. In a large pot, melt the butter on high heat.

2. Put in the carrots, celery, onion, and garlic and sauté until slightly softened two to three minutes.

3. Pour the broth and clam juice, then bring it to its boiling point.

4. Reduce the heat and cook until the carrots are soft, three to five minutes.

5. Mix in the clams and their juices, thyme, salt, and pepper, heat through for two to three minute , before you serve.

Nutritional Info: Calories: 156 , Total Fat: 7g , Total Carbohydrates: 7g , Sugar: 3g , Fiber: 1g , Protein: 14g , Sodium: 981mg

10.   COCONUT CASHEW SOUP WITH BUTTERNUT SQUASH

Time To Prepare: ten minutes **Time to Cook:** twenty minutes **Yield:** Servings 6

Ingredients:

- ½ tsp. salt

- ¾ cup toasted cashews

- 1 (14-ounce) can full-fat coconut milk

- 1 cup mung bean sprouts

- 1 small butternut squash, halved, diced

- 1 small Napa cabbage, shredded

- 1 white onion, diced

- 1½ tbsp. Ginger, peeled and minced

- 2 carrots, chopped

- 2 cups green beans, trimmed

- 2 red chili peppers, seeded and diced

- 2 tbsp. coconut oil

- 3 cups vegetable broth

- 3 garlic cloves, peeled and minced

- 4 tablespoons toasted coconut shavings

- Freshly ground black pepper

Directions:

1. In a huge soup pot on moderate heat, melt the coconut oil.

2. Place the cashews and sauté for a couple of minutes. Take off from the pan and save for later.

3. Place the pepper , garlic, and onion, and sauté for minimum 6 minutes. Then put the ginger and carrots, and sauté for minimum 3 minutes, or until the carrots and squash start to become tender.

4. Stir in the cabbage, green beans, broth, coconut milk, and salt, flavor with pepper. Simmer for fifteen minutes. Remove the heat.

5. Mix in the bean sprouts and coconut shavings.

6. Pour into soup bowls and serve instantly.

Nutritional Info: Calories: 340 , Total Fat: 25g , Saturated Fat: 20g , Cholesterol: 0mg , Carbohydrates: 23g , Fiber: 5g , Protein: 7g

11. COCONUT CURRIED BAN-APPLE SOUP

Time To Prepare: ten minutes

Time to Cook: 10-fifteen minutes **Yield:** Servings 4

Ingredients:

- ¼ cup toasted coconut, for decoration

- 1 big potato 1 Granny Smith apple

- 1 celery heart

- 1 cup coconut milk

- 1 ripe banana

- 1 sweet onion

- 1 teaspoon curry powder

- 1 teaspoon salt

- 2 cups Basic Vegetable Stock or low-sodium canned vegetable stock

- 2 tablespoons chopped fresh cilantro, for decoration

Directions:

1. Place the vegetable stock in a soup pot.

2. Peel the banana and potato, cut them, and place them in the soup pot. Core the apple, cut it, and put in it to the soup pot. Cut the celery heart and onion and put in them to the soup pot.

3. Put the soup to it boiling point, then reduce the heat and simmer for ten to fifteen minutes. Put in the coconut milk, curry powder, and salt.

4. Place the hot soup in a blender and purée.

5. Serve the soup hot. Decorate using toasted coconut and cilantro.

Nutritional Info: Calories: 344 , Fat: 19 g , Protein: 6 g , Sodium: 886 mg , Fiber: 7 g , Carbohydrates: 40 g

12.   CREAM OF MUSHROOM SOUP

Time To Prepare: twenty minutes

Time to Cook: thirty minutes **Yield:** Servings 6

Ingredients:

- 5 cups mushrooms (cut)

- 1 tablespoon sherry

- 3 tablespoons butter

- 3 tablespoons flour

- 1 cup half-and-half

- Salt

- Ground black pepper

- 1½ cups chicken broth

- ½ cup onion (chopped) • 1/8 teaspoon dried thyme

Directions:

1. Cook mushrooms with onion and thyme in the broth until soft. Puree the mixture. Whisk some flour in a pan of melted butter. Put in half-and-half, vegetable puree, and seasoning. Boil until it becomes thick.

2. Put in sherry.

Nutritional Info: Calories: 148 kcal , Carbohydrates: 8.6 g , Fat: 11 g , Protein: 4 g

13. CREAMY & CULTURE TOMATO SAUCE

Time To Prepare: ten minutes

Time to Cook: fifteen-twenty minutes **Yield:** Servings 6

Ingredients:

- ⅛ teaspoon dried thyme

- ⅛ teaspoon freshly ground black pepper

- ¼ cup tomato paste

- ¼ teaspoon chili powder

- ½ cup plain whole-milk yogurt

- ½ teaspoon salt

- 1 small onion, chopped

- 1 tablespoon ghee

- 1 teaspoon dried basil

- 1 teaspoon dried oregano

- 2 (14-ounce) cans diced tomatoes with their juice

- 2 cups vegetable broth • 3 garlic cloves, chopped

Directions:

1. In a huge soup pot on moderate heat, melt the ghee.

2. Place the onion and garlic, and sauté for five minutes.

3. Stir in the basil, oregano, salt, chili powder, pepper, and thyme.

4. Place the tomatoes, broth, and tomato paste, and stir until blended. Heat to a simmer, turn the heat to low, and cook for five to ten minutes. Take away the pot from the heat. With an immersion blender (or in batches in a standard blender), purée the mixture in the pot until you have the desired consistency.

5. Put in the yogurt. Blend for a minute more. Serve instantly.

Nutritional Info: Calories: 157 , Total Fat: 6g , Saturated Fat: 3g , Cholesterol: 3mg , Carbohydrates: 25g , Fiber: 13g , Protein: 8g

14. CREAMY BROCCOLI SOUP

Time To Prepare: fifteen minutes

Time to Cook: 4 hours **Yield:** Servings 7

Ingredients:

- ¼ teaspoon ground black pepper

- ½ teaspoon paprika powder

- ½ teaspoon salt

- ⅔ cup heavy whipping cream • 1 pinch cayenne pepper

- 1 red onion, roughly chopped

- 1 tablespoon olive oil

- 2 cups chicken broth

- 20 ounces (567 g) broccoli, cut into stalks and florets

- 3 garlic cloves, chopped

- 3 tablespoons butter

- ounces (99 g) Cheddar cheese, shredded

Directions:

1. Warm 1 tablespoon of butter and olive oil in a deep cooking pan, then fry the broccoli stalks and chopped onion on moderate heat for five minutes until soft.

2. Put in the garlic and keep frying for a couple of minutes until mildly browned, then drizzle with cayenne pepper, paprika, salt, and ground black pepper. Cook for another one minutes.

3. Pour over the chicken broth. Cover the lid and leave to simmer for five minutes.

4. Take away the cooked vegetables from the deep cooking pan to a food processor and process. Lightly ladle the soup into the food processor while processing until creamy.

5. Melt the rest of the butter in the deep cooking pan, and fry the broccoli florets for five minutes until tender and soft.

6. Pour the soup from the food processor into the deep cooking pan. Blend to mix thoroughly. If the soup is too thick, you can put in some water to make it thinner.

7. Bring the soup to its boiling point, then reduce the heat and bring to a simmer using low heat for about three minutes.

8. Put in the Cheddar cheese and heavy whipping cream and cook for a couple of minutes more until the cheese melts.

9. Take away the soup from the deep cooking pan and serve warm.

Nutritional Info: calories: 266 , total fat: 23g , net carbs: 7g , fiber: 3g , protein: 8g

15. CREAMY CELERY AND CHICKEN BROTH

Time To Prepare: five minutes

Time to Cook: twenty minutes **Yield:** Servings 4

Ingredients:

- ¼ cup celery, chopped

- ½ cup coconut cream

- 1 onion, chopped

- 2 chicken breasts, chopped

- 3 tablespoons butter

- 4 cups water

- From The Cupboard:

- Salt and freshly ground black pepper, to taste

Directions:

1. Place the butter in a deep cooking pan, and melt on moderate heat.

2. Put in and sauté the celery and onion for about three minutes or until the onion is translucent.

3. Put in the chicken, salt, black pepper, and water, and simmer for fifteen minutes. Keep stirring during the simmering.

4. Mix in the coconut cream. Pour the soup in a big container and serve warm.

Nutritional Info: calories: 398 , total fat: 24.4g , net carbs: 5.9g , protein: 29.3g

16.   CREAMY LEEK SOUP

Time To Prepare: two minutes

Time to Cook: 8 minutes **Yield:** Servings 4

Ingredients:

- ½ cup heavy cream

- ½ cup Monterey-Jack cheese, shredded

- ½ cup tomato purée

- ½ pound chorizo, cut

- 1 bay leaf

- 1 cup leeks, chopped

- 1 green chili, deseeded and finely chopped

- 1 tablespoon sesame oil

- 2 chicken bouillon cubes

- 2 cloves garlic, minced

- 4 cups water

Directions:

1.   Push the "Sauté" button to heat up your Instant Pot. Once hot, heat the oil and sauté the leeks until soft.

2. Now, mix in chorizo, garlic, and green chili; carry on cooking until aromatic. Next, put in water, tomato puree, heavy cream, bouillon cubes, and bay leaf.

3. Secure the lid. Choose "Manual" mode and High pressure; cook for about six minutes. Once cooking is complete, use a natural pressure release; cautiously remove the lid.

4. Next, press the "Sauté" button and put in the cheese; allow it to simmer until the cheese is melted and thoroughly heated.

Nutritional Info: 428 Calories , 36g Fat , 6.1g Total Carbs , 18.9g Protein , 2.1g Sugars

17.   CREAMY PARSNIP SOUP

Time To Prepare: twenty-five minutes

Time to Cook: 60 minutes **Yield:** Servings 10

Ingredients:

- 1 big onion (diced)

- 1 cup whole milk

- 1 tablespoon brown sugar

- 1 tablespoon butter

- 1 tablespoon olive oil

- 1 teaspoon ground ginger

- ½ teaspoon ground allspice

- ½ teaspoon ground cardamom

- ½ teaspoon ground nutmeg

- 1/4 teaspoon cayenne pepper

- 2 pounds parsnips (peeled, cut)

- 3 carrots (peeled, cut)

- 3 cloves garlic (minced)

- 3 stalks celery (diced)

- 4 cups chicken stock

- Ground black pepper

- Salt

Directions:

1. Preheat your oven to 425 F.

2. Toss the parsnips and carrots with oil and seasoning in a container. Put them over a baking sheet.

3. Roast in oven until for half an hour

4. Cook the onion and celery in oil till golden brown, approximately seven minutes. Put in butter, brown sugar, garlic, and the parsnips and carrots, cooking for about ten minutes.

5. Season and stir. Put in the chicken stock to its boiling point until soft.

6. Puree the soup.

7. Put in milk and cream and simmer some more before you serve with seasoning.

Nutritional Info: Calories: 187 kcal , Carbohydrates: 24 g , Fat: 9 g , Protein: 3 g

18.   CREAMY PUMPKIN PUREE SOUP

Time To Prepare: ten minutes

Time to Cook: forty-five minutes **Yield:** Servings 3

Ingredients:

- 1 cup Heavy Cream

- 1 cup Pumpkin puree

- 2 cups Chicken broth

- 2 tbsp. Olive oil

- 4-5 Garlic cloves

- Salt and black pepper to taste

Directions:

1. In the Instant Pot, put in all ingredients.

2. Secure the lid and cook for forty minutes on Meat/Stew mode on High. When ready, press Cancel and do a quick pressure release.

3. Move to a blender and blend thoroughly. Pour into serving bowls to serve.

Nutritional Info: Calories 465 , Protein: 15.4g , Carbs: 6.2g , Fat: 43.5g

19.   CREAMY TURKEY SOUP

Time To Prepare: fifteen minutes

Time to Cook: 4 hours **Yield:** Servings 7

Ingredients:

- 1 carrot, chopped

- 1 cup cream cheese

- 1 pound turkey breast, cubed

- 1 stalk celery, chopped

- 1 teaspoon freshly chopped rosemary

- 3 cloves garlic, chopped

- 5 cups chicken broth • Salt & black pepper, to taste

Directions:

1. Put in all the ingredients minus the cream cheese to the base of a slow cooker.

2. Cook on high for 4 hours.

3. Mix in the cream cheese until well blended.

Nutritional Info: Calories: 216 , Carbohydrates: 6g , Fiber: 1g Net , Carbohydrates: 5g , Fat: 14g , Protein: 17g

20. CREAMY TURMERIC CAULIFLOWER SOUP

Time To Prepare: ten minutes

Time to Cook: fifteen minutes **Yield:** Servings 4

Ingredients:

- ¼ cup finely chopped fresh cilantro

- ¼ teaspoon freshly ground black pepper

- ¼ teaspoon ground cumin

- ½ teaspoon salt

- 1 (1¼-inch) piece fresh ginger, peeled and cut

- 1 cup full-fat coconut milk

- 1 garlic clove, peeled

- 1 leek, white part only, thinly cut

- 1½ teaspoons turmeric

- 2 tablespoons extra-virgin olive oil

- 3 cups cauliflower florets

- 3 cups vegetable broth

Directions:

1. In a large pot, heat the oil on high heat.

2. Put in the leek, and sauté until it just starts to brown, three to four minutes. 3. Put in the cauliflower, garlic, ginger, turmeric, salt, pepper, and cumin and sauté to lightly toast the spices, one to two minutes.

4. Pour the broth then bring to its boiling point. Reduce the heat and cook until the cauliflower is soft about five minutes. 6. Use an immersion blender to purée the soup in the pot until the desired smoothness is achieved. 7. Stir in the coconut milk and cilantro, heat through, before you serve.

Nutritional Info: Calories: 264 , Total Fat: 23g , Total Carbohydrates: 12g , Sugar: 5g , Fiber: 4g , Protein: 7g , Sodium: 900mg

21.   CROCK-POT TURKEY TACO SOUP

Time To Prepare: ten minutes

Time to Cook: 4 hours **Yield:** Servings 6

Ingredients:

- 1 cup canned diced tomatoes (no sugar added)

- 1 cup whipped cream cheese

- 1 pound ground turkey

- 1 tablespoon chili powder

- 1 teaspoon cumin 1 teaspoon garlic powder

- 1 teaspoon onion powder

- 1 yellow onion, chopped

- 5 cups chicken bone broth (you can also use regular chicken broth)

  Directions:

1. Put in all the ingredients to the base of a Crock-Pot minus the cream cheese and cover with the chicken broth.

2. Set on high and cook for 4 hours putting in in the cream cheese at the 3.5 hour mark.

3. Stir thoroughly before you serve.

Nutritional Info: Calories: 335, Carbohydrates: 6g, Fiber: 1gNet , Carbohydrates: 5g, Fat: 23g, Protein: 28g

22. DETOX CABBAGE SOUP

Time To Prepare: ten minutes

Time to Cook: thirty-five minutes **Yield:** Servings 4 **Ingredients:**

- 1 tbs. freshly grated ginger root

- 2 big carrot

- 1 cup whole canned tomatoes with juice

- 1 whole head of cabbage

- 1 tbs. freshly grated turmeric root

- 3 celery stalks with leaves

- Enough water to immerse the vegetables

- 2 medium Russet potatoes

- Sea salt & black pepper to taste

- ½ medium onion

- 1/4 cup extra virgin olive oil

Directions:

1. Heat the oil in a large pot on moderate heat for a couple of minutes.

2. Put in the celery, onions, ginger, carrots & turmeric, then sauté on medium until translucent. Sprinkle with salt & pepper to taste.

3. With the heat still on moderate, dice the potatoes & generally slash the cabbage at that point put in to the pot alongside the whole

tomatoes & juice. 4. While they cook, break separated the tomatoes using a fork or blade. Fill the pot with sufficient water to simply cover the cabbage.

5. Cover with a top & heat to the point of boiling. When bubbling, evacuate the top & cook for around thirty minutes or until the potatoes & cabbage are fork delicate. Put in the ice chest for as long as 5 days & in the cooler for as long as three months.

Nutritional Info: Calories: 359 kcal , Protein: 10.85 g , Fat: 12.68 g , Carbohydrates: 54.94 g

23.   FENNEL AND PEAR SOUP

Time To Prepare: fifteen minutes

Time to Cook: twenty minutes **Yield:** Servings 4

Ingredients:

- ⅛ Teaspoon ground nutmeg

- ¼ cup freshly squeezed lemon juice

- ¼ cup honey

- ¼ teaspoon freshly ground black pepper

- 1 teaspoon finely chopped fresh tarragon

- 1 teaspoon salt

- 2 fennel bulbs, trimmed and slice into ½-inch dice

- 2 shallots, halved

- 2 tablespoons extra-virgin olive oil

- 4 cups vegetable broth

- 4 pears, cored and slice into ½-inch dice

Directions:

1. In a large pot, heat the oil on high heat.

2. Put in the pears, fennel, and shallots, and sauté until the pears and fennel barely start to brown, approximately five minutes.

3. Pour the broth, then bring to its boiling point.

4. Reduce the heat to a simmer, then cook, once in a while stirring, until the fennel is soft, 5 to 8 minutes.

5. Stir in the lemon juice, honey, salt, pepper, and nutmeg.

6. Use an immersion blender to purée the soup in the pot until the desired smoothness is achieved.

7. Drizzle with the tarragon before you serve.

Nutritional Info: Calories: 328 , Total Fat: 9g , Total Carbohydrates: 60g , Sugar: 39g , Fiber: 10g , Protein: 7g , Sodium: 1413mg

24. FRENCH CARAMELIZED ONION SOUP

Time To Prepare: five minutes

Time to Cook: ten minutes **Yield:** Servings 4

Ingredients:

- ½ stick butter, softened

- 4 cups chicken stock ½ teaspoon dried basil

- Kosher salt and ground black pepper, to taste

- ½ cup Swiss cheese, freshly grated

- 3/4 pound yellow onions, cut

Directions:

1. Push the "Sauté" button to heat up your Instant Pot. Once hot, melt the butter and sauté the onions until caramelized and soft.

2. Put in chicken stock, basil, salt, and black pepper.

3. Secure the lid. Choose "Manual" mode and High pressure; cook for about ten minutes. Once cooking is complete, use a quick pressure release; cautiously remove the lid.

4. Ladle the soup into separate bowls and top with grated cheese. Enjoy!

Nutritional Info: 228 Calories , 18g Fat , 5.3g Total Carbs , 10.5g Protein , 3.5g Sugars

25. GARLIC AND LENTIL SOUP

Time To Prepare: fifteen minutes

Time to Cook: fifteen minutes **Yield:** Servings 4

Ingredients:

- ¼ cup chopped walnuts (not necessary)

- ¼ teaspoon freshly ground black pepper

- 1 (fifteen-ounce) can lentils, drained and washed

- 1 small white onion, cut into ¼-inch dice

- 1 tablespoon minced or grated orange zest

- 1 teaspoon ground cinnamon

- 1 teaspoon salt

- 2 garlic cloves, thinly cut

- 2 medium carrots, thinly cut

- 2 tablespoons extra-virgin olive oil

- 2 tablespoons finely chopped fresh flat-leaf parsley

- 3 cups vegetable broth

Directions:

1. In a large pot, heat the oil using high heat.

2. Put in the carrots, onion, and garlic and sauté until tender, five to seven minutes.

3. Place the cinnamon, salt, and pepper and stir to uniformly coat the vegetables, one to two minutes.

4. Pour the broth then bring to its boiling point.

5. Reduce the heat to a simmer, put in the lentils and cook until they are thoroughly heated about one minute.

6. Mix in the orange zest and serve, sprinkled with the walnuts (if using) and parsley.

Nutritional Info: Calories: 201 , Total Fat: 8g , Total Carbohydrates 22g , Sugar: 4g , Fiber: 8g , Protein: 11g , Sodium: 1178mg

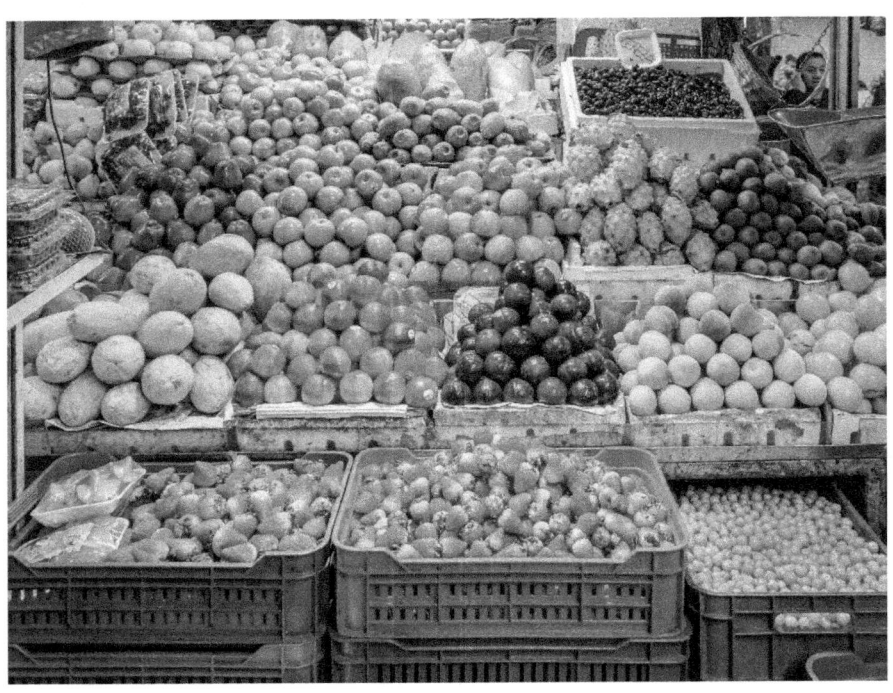

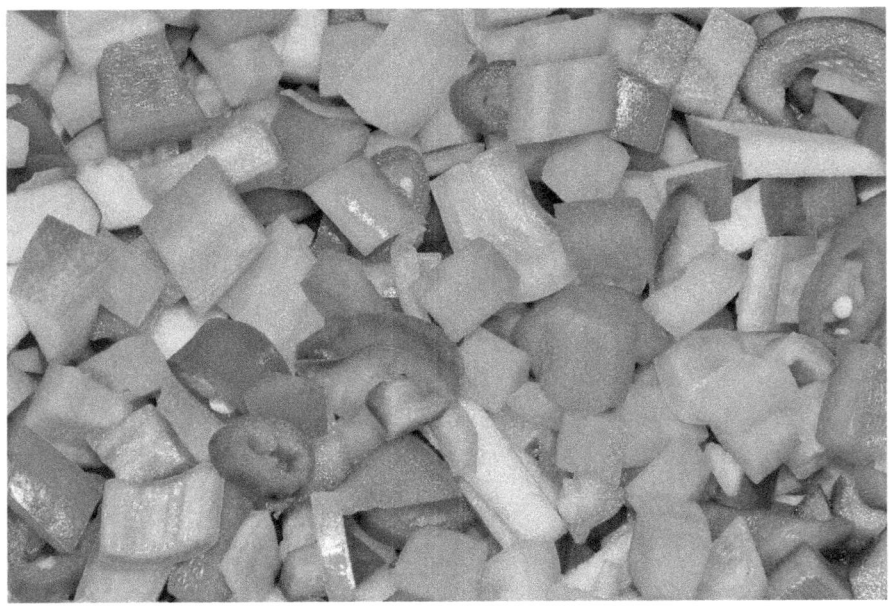

26.   GARLIC MUSHROOM & BEEF SOUP

Time To Prepare: ten minutes

Time to Cook: forty minutes **Yield:** Servings 6

Ingredients:

- ½ cup heavy cream

- ½ cup whipped cream cheese

- 1 pound beef chuck, cubed

- 1 tablespoon coconut oil, for cooking

- 1 yellow onion, chopped 1½ cups cremini mushrooms

- 2 cloves garlic, chopped

- 6 cups beef broth • Salt & pepper, to taste

Directions:

1. Put in the coconut oil to a frying pan and brown the beef.

2. Once cooked, put in the beef to the base of a stockpot with all of the ingredients minus the heavy cream. Mix thoroughly.

3. Heat to a simmer and whisk again until the cream cheese is mixed uniformly into the soup. 4. Cook for half an hour

5. Warm the heavy cream, and then put in to the soup.

Nutritional Info: Calories: 315, Carbohydrates: 5g, Fiber: 1gNet , Carbohydrates: 4g, Fat: 19g, Protein: 30g

27. GARLICKY CHICKEN SOUP

Time To Prepare: ten minutes

Time to Cook: fifteen minutes **Yield:** Servings 6 **Ingredients:**

- ¼ teaspoon black pepper

- ½ cup whipped cream cheese

- 1 tablespoon butter for cooking

- 1 teaspoon salt 1 teaspoon thyme

- 2 boneless, skinless chicken breasts

- 3 cloves garlic, chopped 4 cups chicken broth

Directions:

1. Preheat a stockpot on moderate heat with the butter.

2. Put in the chicken and brown until completely thoroughly cooked. Turn off the heat.

3. Shred the chicken and put in it back to the stockpot together with the rest of the ingredients minus the cream cheese.

4. Heat to a simmer.

5. Put in in the cream cheese and whisk until there are no more clumps.

6. Simmer for about ten minutes before you serve.

Nutritional Info: Calories: 128 , Carbohydrates: 2g , Fiber: 0g Net , Carbohydrates: 2g , Fat: 6g , Protein: 16g

28. GOLDEN CHICKPEA AND VEGETABLE SOUP

Time To Prepare: fifteen minutes

Time to Cook: twenty minutes

Yield: Servings 6 **Ingredients:**

- 1 ½ cup Diced celery

- 1 ½ cup Sliced leeks

- 1 cup cooked chickpeas

- 1 cup diced carrots

- 1 cup Torn curly kale leaves

- 1 tbsp. Grated ginger

- 2 cloves minced garlic

- 2 cups Cauliflower florets

- 2 tbsp. Curry powder

- 2 tbsp. Minced organic parsley

- 2 tsp. Coconut oil • 4 cups Bone broth

Directions:

1. Warm the coconut oil in a pot and put in the garlic and ginger. Sauté for one minute before you put in the turmeric and curry powder and sautéing for one more minute.

2. Throw in celery, leeks, carrots, and cauliflower, continuously stirring for approximately one minute.

3. Put in the bone broth and chickpeas. Cover the pot and leave to boil. Reduce the heat and allow it to simmer for minimum fifteen minutes.

4. Turn off heat and put in parsley and kale, leaving the heat to cook the leaves.

5. Drizzle salt and pepper.

6. Serve.

Nutritional Info: Calories: 142 kcal , Protein: 8.64 g , Fat: 4.79 g , Carbohydrates: 17.57 g

29. GREEK SPLIT PEA SOUP

Time To Prepare: fifteen minutes

Time to Cook: 2 hours **Yield:** Servings 6

Ingredients:

- 1 pinch dried marjoram

- 1 potato (diced)

- 1½ pounds ham bone

- 2 onions (cut)

- 2 quarts cold water

- 2-1/4 cups dried split peas

- 3 carrots, (chopped)

- 3 stalks celery (chopped)

- Ground black pepper

- Salt

Directions:

1. Simmer the peas in a pot for a couple of minutes and then soak for an hour.

2. Put in ham bone, onion, marjoram, and seasoning.

3. Boil for 1½hours.

4. Remove bone and meat. Put in the meat (diced) to the soup.

5. Put the rest of the vegetables and cook until soft.

Nutritional Info: Calories: 310 kcal , Carbohydrates: 58 g , Fat: 20 g , Protein: 2 g

30. GREEN BLAST SOUP

Time To Prepare: ten minutes **Time to Cook:** twenty minutes **Yield:** Servings 4

Ingredients:

- ¼ cup chopped cashews (not necessary)

- ¼ cup extra-virgin olive oil

- ¼ teaspoon freshly ground black pepper

- 1 bunch Swiss chard, crudely chopped

- 1 fen el bulb, trimmed and thinly cut

- 1 garlic clove, peeled

- 1 teaspoon salt

- 2 leeks, white parts only, thinly cut

- 2 tablespoons apple cider vinegar

- 3 cups vegetable broth

- 4 cups crudely chopped kale

- 4 cups crudely chopped mustard greens

Directions:

1. In a large pot, heat the oil on high heat.

2. Put in the leeks, fennel, and garlic and sauté until tender, for approximately five minutes.

3. Put in the Swiss chard, kale, and mustard greens and sauté until the greens wilt, two to three minutes.

4. Pour the broth then bring to its boiling point.

5. Reduce the heat to a simmer and cook until the vegetables are completely tender and soft about five minutes.

6. Mix in the vinegar, salt, pepper, and cashews (if using).

7. Use an immersion blender to purée the soup in the pot until the desired smoothness is achieved before you serve.

Nutritional Info: Calories: 238 , Total Fat: 14g , Total Carbohydrates: 22g , Sugar: 4g , Fiber: 6g , Protein: 9g , Sodium: 1294mg

31.   GUT-HEALING BONE BROTH

Time To Prepare: fifteen minutes

Time to Cook: 8 to one day **Yield:** Servings 4

Ingredients:

- 1 medium onion, chopped

- 1 tablespoon apple cider vinegar

- 2 bay leaves 2 celery stalks, chopped

- 2 pou ds beef marrow bones

- 3 medium carrots, chopped

- 4 garlic cloves • Filtered water, to cover

Directions:

1.   In a 6-quart slow cooker, mix the bones, garlic, carrots, celery, onion, bay leaves, and vinegar. Cover with filtered water. Set the cooker on low and simmer for minimum 8 hours and up to one day.

2.   Skim off and discard any foam that forms on the surface. Ladle the broth through a fine-mesh sieve or cheesecloth to strain out the solids. Pour into airtight glass containers. The broth can be placed in the fridge for maximum one week; just boil it again before use. To freeze, let the broth fully cool and then fill jars up to an inch below the top to allow for expansion, and keep for four to 5 months.

Nutritional Info: Calories: 40 , Total Fat: 0g , Saturated Fat: 0g , Cholesterol: 0mg , Carbohydrates: 5g , Fiber: 0g , Protein: 6g

32.   HAMBURGER & TOMATO SOUP

Time To Prepare: ten minutes

Time to Cook: 4 hours **Yield:** Servings 6

Ingredients:

- ½ cup beef broth

- ½ cup no-sugar added marinara sauce

- ½ cup shredded cheddar cheese

- 1 pound lean ground beef

- 1 yellow onion, chopped

- 2 cloves garlic, chopped

- Salt & pepper, to taste

Directions:

1. Put i all the ingredients to a slow cooker minus the shredded cheese and cook on high for 4 hours.

2. Mix in the cheese before you serve.

Nutritional Info: Calories: 209 , Carbohydrates: 5g , Fiber: 1g Net , Carbohydrates: 4g , Fat: 9g , Protein: 26g

33.   HARVEST STEW

Time To Prepare: fifteen minutes

Time to Cook: 60 minutes **Yield:** Servings 6

Ingredients:

- ¼ cup flour

- ½ cup cut carrots

- ½ cup diced celery

- ¾ cup diced onions

- 1 bay leaf

- 1 leek, cleaned and diced

- 1 potato, peeled and diced

- 1 pound stewing beef cubes

- 2 cups diced zucchini

- 2 tablespoons olive oil

- 2 tablespoons Worcestershire sauce

- 2 tomatoes, chopped

- 3 sprigs fresh thyme

- 3 turnips, diced

- 4 cups low-sodium beef broth

• 6 garlic cloves, peeled • Salt and pepper, to taste

Directions:

1. Brown the beef cubes in olive oil. Dust the flour on the meat and stir to coat and spread.

2. Put in the onions, carrots, celery, leek, garlic, zucchini, potato, turnips, tomatoes, bay leaf, thyme sprigs, and beef broth. Put to its boiling point, then reduce the heat and simmer for 60 minutes.

3. Take away the bay leaf and thyme sprigs. Put in the Worcestershire sauce, salt, and pepper. Serve hot.

Nutritional Info: Calories: 254 , Fat: 9.5 g , Protein: 20 g , Sodium: 514 mg , Fiber: 3.5 g , Carbohydrates: 22 g

34.   HEARTY ROOT VEGETABLE SOUP

Time To Prepare: five minutes

Time to Cook: ten minutes **Yield:** Servings 4

Ingredients:

- 1 bay leaf

- 1 carrot, cut

- 1 celery, diced

- 1 garlic clove, minced

- 1 parsnip, cut

- 1 tablespoon fresh parsley, roughly chopped

- 1 teaspoon fresh sage

- 2 cups cauliflower, cut into little florets

- 4 cups chicken stock

- 4 tablespoons olive oil

- Kosher salt and freshly ground black pepper, to taste

Directions:

1. Simply drop all of the above ingredients into your Instant Pot.

2. Secure the lid. Choose "Manual" mode and High pressure; cook for about ten minutes. Once cooking is complete, use a natural pressure release; cautiously remove the lid.

3. Taste, calibrate the seasonings and serve instantly. Enjoy!

Nutritional Info: 190 Calories , 15.6g Fat , 6.1g Total Carbs , 6.7g Protein , 2.6g Sugars

35.   HUNGARIAN LENTIL SOUP

Time To Prepare: fifteen minutes

Time to Cook: 2 hours **Yield:** Servings 8

Ingredients:

- 7 Cups Chicken Stock

- 3 Carrots (Diced)

- 2 Stalks Celery (Diced)

- 1 Teaspoon Garlic (Minced)

- 2 Bay Leaves

- 1 Sprig Fresh Parsley (Chopped)

- 2 Tablespoons Olive Oil

- 2 Large Onions (Cubed)

- Salt

- Ground Black Pepper

- 1½ Cups Lentils (Soaked, Rinsed, Drained)

- ½ Teaspoon Paprika

- ½ Cup Grated Parmesan Cheese

- 3½ Cups Crushed Tomatoes

- 3/4 Cup White Wine

Directions:

1. Sauté onions in oil until shiny and put in garlic, paprika, celery, and carrots, cooking for about ten minutes.

2. Mix in tomatoes, chicken stock, lentils, bay leaves, seasoning, and wine to boil.

3. Cook until the lentils are soft.

4. Top with parsley and Parmesan before you serve.

Nutritional Info: Calories: 258 kcal , Carbohydrates: 34 g , Fat: 6 g , Protein: 14 g

36.　　ITALIAN BEEF SOUP

Time To Prepare: ten minutes

Time to Cook: 4 hours **Yield:** Servings 6

Ingredients:

- ½ cup diced tomatoes

- ½ cup shredded mozzarella cheese

- 1 cup beef broth

- 1 cup heavy cream

- 1 pound lean ground beef

- 1 tablespoon Italian seasoning

- 1 yellow onion, chopped

- 2 cloves garlic, chopped

- Salt & pepper, to taste

Directions:

1.　　Put in all the ingredients to a slow cooker minus the heavy cream and mozzarella cheese. Cook on high for 4 hours.

2.　　Warm the heavy cream, and then put in the warmed cream and cheese to the soup. Stir thoroughly before you serve.

Nutritional Info: Calories: 241 , Carbohydrates: 4g , Fiber: 1g Net , Carbohydrates: 3g , Fat: 14g , Protein: 25g

37. ITALIAN MODENA SOUP

Time To Prepare: two minutes

Time to Cook: 8 minutes

Yield: Servings 4

Ingredients:

- ½ cup Parmigiano-Reggiano cheese, shaved

- ½ teaspoon crushed chili

- 1 cup water

- 1 onion, chopped

- 1 tablespoon Italian seasonings

- 16 ounces Cotechino di Modena, cut

- 2 cups tomatoes, purée

- 2 tablespoons olive oil

- 3 cups roasted vegetable broth

- Sea salt and ground black pepper, to taste

Directions:

1. Push the "Sauté" button to heat up your Instant Pot. Once hot, heat the oil and sauté the onions until soft and translucent.

2. Now, put in the sausage and cook an additional three minutes,

3. Mix in tomatoes, broth, water, sea salt, black pepper, crushed chili, and Italian seasonings.

4. Secure the lid. Choose "Manual" mode and High pressure; cook for five minutes. Once cooking is complete, use a quick pressure release; cautiously remove the lid.

5. Top with shaved Parmigiano-Reggiano cheese and serve warm

Nutritional Info: 340 Calories , 27.9g Fat , 5g Total Carbs , 14.1g Protein , 2.6g Sugars

38. ITALIAN SUMMER SQUASH SOUP

Time To Prepare: ten minutes

Time to Cook: fifteen minutes **Yield:** Servings 4

Ingredients:

- ½ cup shredded carrot

- 1 cup shredded yellow squash

- 1 cup shredded zucchini

- 1 garlic clove, minced

- 1 small red onion, thinly cut

- 1 tablespoon finely chopped fresh chives

- 1 teaspoon salt

- 2 tablespoons finely chopped fresh basil

- 2 tablespoons pine nuts

- 3 cups vegetable broth

- 3 tablespoons extra-virgin olive oil

Directions:

1. In a large pot, heat the oil using high heat.

2. Put in the onion and garlic and sauté until tender, five to seven minutes.

3. Put in the zucchini, yellow squash, and carrot and sauté until tender, one to two minutes.

4. Pour the broth and salt then bring to its boiling point.

5. Reduce the heat and cook until the vegetables are soft, one to two minutes.

6. Mix in the basil and chives and serve, sprinkled with the pine nuts.

Nutritional Info: Calories: 172 , Total Fat: 15g , Total Carbohydrates: 6g , Sugar: 3g , Fiber: 2g , Protein: 5g , Sodium: 1170mg

39.　KUMARA & CHICKPEA SOUP

Time To Prepare: twenty-five minutes

Time to Cook: thirty-five minutes **Yield:** Servings 6

Ingredients:

- 1 bay leaf

- 1 onion (chopped)

- 1 teaspoon dried basil

- 1 tomato (chopped)

- ½ teaspoon dried thyme

- 1/4 teaspoon paprika

- 2 cloves garlic (minced)

- 2 cups kumara (peeled, chopped)

- 2 tablespoons olive oil

- 200g garbanzo beans

- 3 cups chicken broth

- Ground black pepper

- Mixed vegetables Salt

Directions:

1. Sauté onion, garlic, and sweet potatoes in oil for five minutes.

2. Put in broth, bay leaf, herbs, and seasoning.

3. Boil until soft.

4. Put in tomato, beans, and chickpeas, simmering some more before you serve.

Nutritional Info: Calories: 197 kcal , Carbohydrates: 30 g , Fat: 6 g , Protein: 7.5 g

40.   LAMB STEW

Time To Prepare: five minutes

Time to Cook: 8 hours **Yield:** Servings 6

Ingredients:

- 1 lamb stock cube

- 1 onion, roughly chopped

- 2 pounds (907 g) boneless lamb, cut into cubes

- 2 tablespoons olive oil, plus more for greasing the frying pan

- 2 teaspoons dried rosemary

- 3 cups water

- 4 garlic cloves, finely chopped

- From the cupboard:

- Salt and freshly ground black pepper, to taste

Directions:

1. Position the lamb into a mildly greased nonstick frying pan, and cook using high heat for a couple of minutes or until browned.

2. Grease a slow cooker with olive oil, then put in the cooked lamb, stock cube, rosemary, onion, garlic, salt, black pepper, and 3 cups of water. Blend to blend well.

3. Place the slow cooker lid on and cook on LOW for eight hours.

4. Take away the cooked lamb stew from the slow cooker and serve warm.

Nutritional Info: calories: 252 , total fat: 9.5g , carbs: 4.9g , protein: 34.9g

41.   LAMB TACO SOUP

Time To Prepare: ten minutes

Time to Cook: 4-6 hours minutes **Yield:** Servings 6

Ingredients:

- ½ teaspoon cayenne pepper 1 cup diced tomatoes

- 1 cup shredded cheddar cheese

- 1 green bell pepper, chopped

- 1 pound ground lamb

- 1 teaspoon ground coriander

- 1 teaspoon ground cumin

- 1 teaspoon paprika

- 1 yellow onion, chopped

- 2 cloves garlic, chopped

- 4 cups beef broth • Salt & pepper, to taste

Directions:

1. Put in all the ingredients to a slow cooker minus the shredded cheese and cook on high for four to 6 hours.

2. Mix in the shredded cheese before you serve.

Nutritional Info: Calories: 265 , Carbohydrates: 6g , Fiber: 1g Net , Carbohydrates: 5g , Fat: 13g , Protein: 30g

42.   LEBANESE LENTIL SOUP

Time To Prepare: fifteen minutes

Time to Cook: 60 minutes **Yield:** Servings 6

Ingredients:

- 1 cup brown lentils

- 1 lemon juiced

- 1 medium onion

- 1 tablespoon olive oil

- 2 medium carrots

- 2 teaspoons cinnamon

- 2 teaspoons cumin

- 3 stalks celery

- 4 cloves garlic

- 4 cups chicken broth low sodium

- 4 cups water

- 8 cups spinach • salt& pepper to taste

Directions:

1.   Over moderate heat, heat oil in a soup pot, Put in & cook carrots, celery & onions until become soft for seven minutes, put in pepper & salt to taste.

2.   Stir cumin, cinnamon & garlic heat it for 30-60 minutes. Put in lentils & heat for a couple of minutes to slightly toast. Pour in the lemon juice, water & chicken broth, then bring the pot to its boiling point. When lentils are soft, decrease the heat to low & simmer, approximately 30-45 minutes.

3.   Before you serve, mix in the spinach, cook until the color is green, now served to put in pepper, lemon juice & salt.

Nutritional Info: Calories: 102 kcal , Protein: 6.33 g , Fat: 4.58 g , Carbohydrates: 11.6 g

43.   LEEK, CHICKEN AND SPINACH SOUP

Time To Prepare: ten minutes

Time to Cook: fifteen minutes **Yield:** Servings 4

Ingredients:

- ¼ teaspoon freshly ground black pepper

- 1 tablespoon thinly cut fresh chives

- 1 teaspoon salt

- 2 cups shredded rotisserie chicken

- 2 leeks, white parts only, thinly cut

- 2 teaspoons grated or minced lemon zest

- 3 tablespoons unsalted butter

- 4 cups baby spinach • 4 cups chicken broth

Directions:

1. In a large pot, melt the butter on high heat.

2. Put in the leeks and sauté until tender and starting to brown, three to five minutes.

3. Put in the spinach, broth, salt, and pepper and bring to its boiling point.

4. Reduce the heat and cook till the spinach wilts, one to two minutes.

5. Place the chicken and cook until warmed through one to two minutes.

6. Drizzle with the chives and lemon zest before you serve.

Nutritional Info: Calories: 256 , Total Fat: 12g , Total Carbohydrates: 9g , Sugar: 3g , Fiber: 2g , Protein: 27g , Sodium: 1483mg

44.   LEMON CHICKEN SOUP

Time To Prepare: ten minutes

Time to Cook: 4 hours **Yield:** Servings 4

Ingredients:

- ¼ cup freshly squeezed lemon juice

- 1 yellow onion, chopped

- 2 boneless, skinless chicken breasts

- 2 cloves garlic, chopped

- 2 tablespoons chives, chopped

- 6 cups chicken broth • Salt & pepper, to taste

Directions:

1. Put in all the ingredients to a slow cooker and cook on high for 4 hours.

2. Once cooked, shred the chicken and stir back into the soup.

Nutritional Info: Calories: 171 , Carbohydrates: 6g , Fiber: 1g Net , Carbohydrates: 5g , Fat: 6g , Protein: 22g

45. MEDITERRANEAN STEW

Time To Prepare: ten minutes

Time to Cook: fifteen minutes **Yield:** Servings 4

Ingredients:

- 1 (19-ounce) can cannellini beans, drained and washed

- 1 (fifteen½-ounce) can chickpeas, drained and washed

- 1 cup Basic Vegetable Stock or low-sodium canned vegetable stock

- 1 teaspoon dried oregano

- 1 teaspoon red pepper, crushed or to taste

- 1½ cups artichoke hearts, quartered

- cups roasted tomatoes

- cloves garlic, crushed and minced

- tablespoons olive oil

- tablespoons grated Par   san cheese

- Chopped Italian parsley, for decoration

- Chopped sun-dried tomatoes, for decoration

- Crumbled feta cheese, for decoration

- Fresh oregano leaves, for decoration

- Freshly ground black pepper, to taste

- Garlic-seasoned croutons, for decoration

- Salt, to taste

Directions:

1.   Warm the olive oil in a huge deep cooking pan on moderate heat and sauté the garlic for two to three minutes or until golden.

2.   Lower the heat to moderate-low. Mix in the chickpeas, cannellini beans, roasted tomatoes, artichoke hearts, stock, Parmesan cheese, crushed red pepper, oregano, salt, and pepper. Cook and stir for approximately ten minutes. Serve in separate bowls, garnishing as you wish.

Nutritional Info: Calories: 445 , Fat: 16 g , Protein: 18 g , Sodium: 530 mg , Fiber: 12 g , Carbohydrates: 61 g

46. MINESTRONE SOUP WITH QUINOA

Time To Prepare: ten minutes **Time to Cook:** twenty minutes **Yield:** Servings 6

Ingredients:

- ½ cup quinoa, washed well

- ½ red bell pepper, diced

- ½ teaspoon salt

- 1 (14 oz.) can cannellini beans, drained and washed well

- 1 (14 oz.) can diced tomatoes with its juice

- 1 bay leaf

- 1 cup packed kal , stem   d and meticulously washed

- 1 medium white onion, diced

- 1 small zucchini, diced

- 1 tablespoon freshly squeezed lemon juice

- tablespoon ghee

- carrots, chopped

- 2 celery stalks, diced

- 2 garlic cloves, minced

- 2 teaspoons dried rosemary

- 2 teaspoons dried thyme

- 5 cups vegetable broth • Freshly ground black pepper

Directions:

1.   In a huge soup pot on moderate heat, put in the ghee, garlic, onion, carrots, and celery, and sauté for about three minutes.

2.   Put in the zucchini and red bell pepper, and sauté for a couple of minutes. 3. Mix in the broth, tomatoes, beans, kale, quinoa, lemon juice, rosemary, thyme, bay leaf, and salt, and flavor with black pepper. Put it to a simmer, reduce the heat temperature, cover, and cook for fifteen minutes, or until the quinoa is cooked. Take away the bay leaf and discard it. Serve hot.

Nutritional Info: Calories: 319 , Total Fat: 5g , Saturated Fat: 2g , Cholesterol: 0mg , Carbohydrates: 42g , Fiber: 9g , Protein: 18g

47.   MOONG DAAL

Time To Prepare: fifteen minutes

Time to Cook: thirty minutes **Yield:** Servings 6

Ingredients:

- ½ Cup Tomatoes (Diced)

- ½ Dried Red Chili Pepper

- ½ Teaspoon Ginger Root (Grated)

- ½ Teaspoon Ground Tur   ric

- 1 Pinch Asafoetida

- 1 Teaspoon Cumin Seed

- Teaspoon Jalapeno (Diced)

- 1/4 Cup Cilantro (Chopped)

- Cloves Garlic (Chopped)

- 2 Teaspoons Vegetable Oil

- 2½ Cups Moong Dal (Rinsed)

- 2½ Cups Water

- 3 Teaspoons Lemon Juice Salt

Directions:

1. Soak daal for thirty minutes before boiling in water with salt until thick.

2. Put in ginger, jalapeno, tomato, lemon juice, and turmeric.

3. Heat cumin seed and red Chile pepper in a pan before you put in asafoetida powder and garlic. Combine with split peas and serve with cilantro.

Nutritional Info: Calories: 330 kcal , Carbohydrates: 57 g , Fat: 3 g , Protein: 21 g

48. MUSHROOM AND THYME SOUP

Time To Prepare: five minutes

Time to Cook: twenty minutes **Yield:** Servings 4

Ingredients: ¼ cup butter

• 12 ounces (340 g) wild mushrooms, chopped

• 2 garlic cloves, minced

• 2 teaspoons thyme leaves

4 cups vegetable broth 5 ounces (142 g) crème fraiche From the cupboard: Salt and freshly round black pepper, to taste

Directions:

1. Place the butter in a deep cooking pan and melt on moderate heat.

2. Put in the minced garlic and cook for a minutes or until aromatic.

3. Put in the chopped mushrooms, and drizzle with salt and black pepper. Stir to blend and cook for about ten minutes or until the mushrooms are soft. 4. Put in the vegetable broth and bring the soup to its boiling point. Stir continuously. Reduce the heat and simmer the soup for about ten minutes or until it becomes slightly thick. Pour the soup in a blender, and pulse until smooth, then fold in the crème fraiche. Move the soup in a big container and top with thyme leaves before you serve.

Nutritional Info: calories: 282 , total fat: 25.1g , net carbs: 6.3g , protein: 7.8g

49. ONION, KALE AND WHITE BEAN SOUP

Time To Prepare: fifteen minutes

Time to Cook: twenty-five minutes **Yield:** Servings 4

Ingredients:

- ⅛ Teaspoon red pepper flakes (not necessary)

- ¼ cup extra-virgin olive oil

- ¼ teaspoon freshly ground black pepper

- 1 (fifteen½-ounce) can white beans, drained and washed

- 1 big onion, thinly cut

- 1 teaspoon finely chopped fresh rosemary

- teaspoon salt

- garlic cloves, thinly cut

- cups stemmed kale leaves cut into ½-inch pieces

- cups vegetable broth

Directions:

1. In a large pot, heat the oil on high heat.

2. Lower the heat to moderate, and put in the onion, garlic, salt, pepper, and red pepper flakes (if using). Sauté until the onion is golden, approximately ten minutes.

3. Put in the kale, and sauté until wilted, one to two minutes.

4. Pour the broth then bring to its boiling point.

5. Lower the heat to simmer, and cook until the kale is tender about five minutes.

6. Put in the beans and rosemary. Cook until the beans are warmed through minimum two to three minutes before you serve.

Nutritional Info: Calories: 285 , Total Fat: 15g , Total Carbohydrates: 28g , Sugar: 3g , Fiber: 9g , Protein: 13g , Sodium: 1368mg

50.   PORK STEW

Time To Prepare: five minutes

Time to Cook: 8 hours **Yield:** Servings 6

Ingredients:

- 1 onion, finely chopped

- 1 teaspoon dried mixed spices (homemade or store-bought)

- 2 pounds (907 g) pork loin, cut into cubes

- 2 tablespoons olive oil

- 3 cups chicken stock

- 4 garlic cloves, crushed

- From the cupboard:

- Salt and freshly ground black pepper, to taste

Directions:

1. Grease the insert of the slow cooker with olive oil.

2. Combine the pork, chicken stock, onion, dried mixed spices, garlic, salt, and black pepper n the slow cooker.

3. Place the slow cooker lid on and cook on LOW for eight hours.

4. Ladle the stew in a big container and serve warm.

Nutritional Info: calories: 381 , total fat: 18.3g , carbs: 9.2g , protein: 42.3g

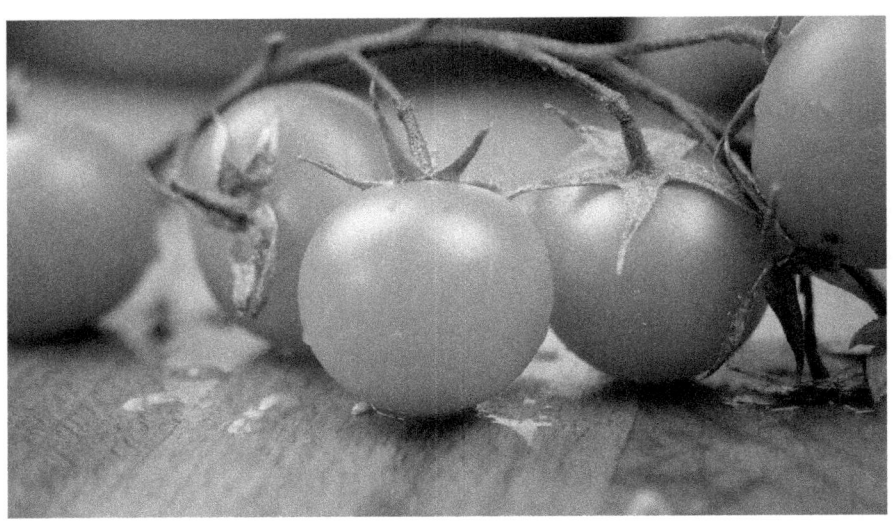

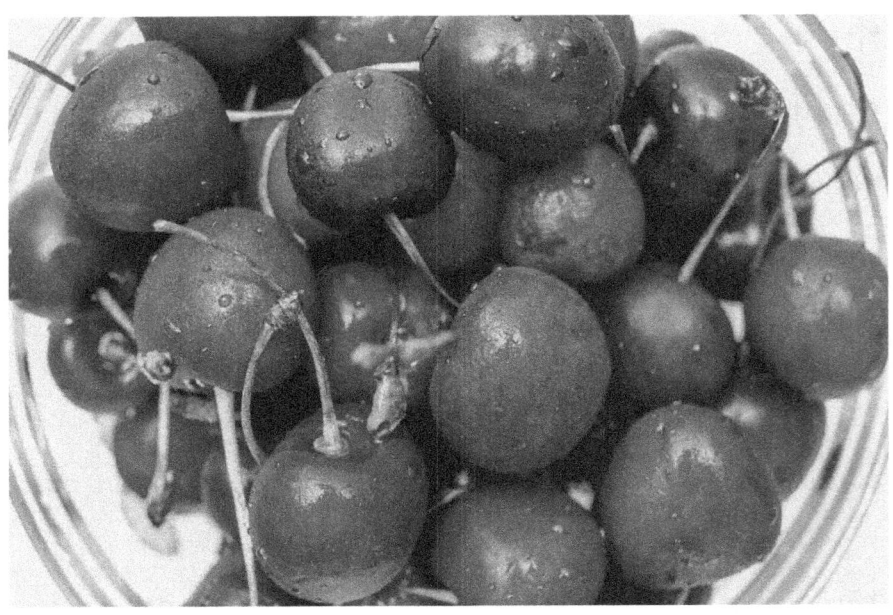

51.   PUMPKIN AND SAUSAGE SOUP

Time To Prepare: five minutes

Time to Cook: 33 minutes **Yield:** Servings 4

Ingredients:

- ½ cup heavy whipping cream

- ½ cup pumpkin puree

- ½ teaspoon dried sage

- ½ teaspoon ground dried thyme

- ½ teaspoon red chili pepper flakes (not necessary)

- 1 garlic clove, minced

- 1 moderate-sized red onion, minced

- 1 pinch salt

- 1 small red bell pepper, diced

- 2 cups chicken broth

- 2 tablespoons butter, melted • pounds (680 g) fresh sausage

Directions:

1. Sauté the sausage in a nonstick frying pan on moderate to high heat for a minutes, then put in the onion and bell pepper. Continue sautéing for about six minutes until the sausage is mildly browned and the onion is translucent. 2. Fold in the chili pepper flakes, thyme, sage, minced

garlic, and salt, then put in the pumpkin puree, chicken broth, and heavy whipping cream.

3.   Reduce the heat and bring them to a simmer using low heat for fifteen minutes or until it becomes thick.

4.   Pour the cooked soup into a big serving container and put in the butter. Stir to mix thoroughly before you serve.

Nutritional Info: calories: 777 , total fat: 70g , net carbs: 7g , fiber: 2g , protein: 27g

52.   PUMPKIN, COCONUT & SAGE SOUP

Time To Prepare: fifteen minutes

Time to Cook: thirty minutes **Yield:** Servings 6

Ingredients:

- 1 cup canned pumpkin

- 1 cup full-fat coconut milk

- 1 teaspoon freshly chopped sage

- 2 cloves garlic, chopped

- 6 cups vegetable broth • Pinch of salt & pepper, to taste

Directions:

1. Put in all the ingredients minus the coconut milk to a stockpot on moderate heat and bring to its boiling point. Reduce to a simmer and cook for half an hour

2. Put in the coconut milk and stir.

Nutritional Info: Calories: 146 , Carbohydrates: 7g , Fiber: 2g Net , Carbohydrates: 5g , Fat: 11g , Protein: 6g

53. QUICK MISO SOUP WITH WILTED GREENS

Time To Prepare: ten minutes **Time to Cook:** five minutes **Yield:** Servings 4

Ingredients:

- ½ teaspoon fish sauce

- 1 cup cut mushrooms

- 1 cup fresh baby spinach, meticulously washed

- 3 cups filtered water

- 3 cups vegetable broth

- 3 tablespoons miso paste

- 4 scallions, cut

Directions:

1. In a huge soup pot on high heat, put in the water, broth, mushrooms, and fish sauce, and bring to its boiling point. Turn off the heat.

2. In a small container, combine the miso paste with ½ cup of heated broth mixture to dissolve the miso. Mix the miso mixture back into the soup.

3. Mix in the spinach and scallions. Serve instantly.

Nutritional Info: Calories: 44 , Total Fat: 0 , Saturated Fat: 0g , Cholesterol: 0mg , Carbohydrates: 8g , Fiber: 1g , Protein: 2g

54.   RED LENTIL DAL

Time To Prepare: ten minutes **Time to Cook:** twenty minutes **Yield:** Servings 6

Ingredients:

- ½ teaspoon salt

- 1 (14-ounce) can unsweetened coconut milk

- 1 bay leaf

- 1 cup red dried lentils, sorted and washed well

- 1 medium tomato, diced

- 1 medium white onion, diced

- 1 tablespoon coconut oil

- 1 teaspoon ground cumin

- 1 teaspoon ground ginger

- 1 teaspoon ground turmeric

- 1 teaspoon mustard seeds

- 1 teaspoon sesame seeds

- 2 garlic cloves, minced

- 2 tablespoons chopped fresh cilantro leaves

- 3 cups vegetable broth • Dash ground cinnamon

Directions:

1. In a huge soup pot using high heat, combine the broth, lentils, and bay leaf, and place to its boiling point. Lessen the heat to moderate-low and simmer for about twenty minutes, or until the lentils are cooked.

2. In the meantime, in a moderate-sized deep cooking pan on moderate heat, sauté the onion and garlic in the coconut oil for a couple of minutes.

3. Put in the tomato, sesame seeds, ginger, cumin, turmeric, mustard seeds, salt, and cinnamon. Cook, regularly stirring, for five minutes. Mix in the coconut milk, then put it to a simmer.

4. Remove and discard the bay leaf. Put in the coconut milk mixture to the lentils together with the cilantro, and stir until blended. Serve alone or over rice if you wish.

Nutritional Info: Calories: 283 , Total Fat: 6g , Saturated Fat: 5g , Cholesterol: 0mg , Carbohydrates: 32g , Fiber: 7g , Protein: 14g

55.   RIBOLLITA

Time To Prepare: forty-five minutes

Time to Cook: 195 minutes **Yield:** Servings 12

Ingredients:

- ½ Cup Olive Oil

- 1 Bunch Kale (Trimmed, Chopped)

- 1 Bunch Swiss Chard (Trimmed, Chopped)

- 1½ Cups Cabbage (Chopped)

- 12½ Inch-Thick Slices French Bread (Toasted)

- 2 Bay Leaves

- 2 Cups Dry Cannellini Beans (Rinsed)

- 2 Onions (Diced)

- 2 Potatoes (Peeled, Cut)

- 3 Carrots (Peeled, Sliced)

- 3 Large Stalks Celery (Chopped)

- 32 Ounce Chicken Broth

- 4 Cups Water

- 4 Sage Leaves

- 5 Cloves Garlic (Minced)

- Grated Parmesan Cheese

- Ground Black Pepper

- Ounce Tomatoes (Diced)

- Salt

Directions:

1. Boil beans in water for minimum five minutes and cool for 70 minutes.

2. Boil beans, garlic, sage leaves, bay leaves, and salt in chicken broth until soft.

3. Discard the leaves from half of the mixture.

4. Combine the remaining until the desired smoothness is achieved. Set aside. 5. Cook onions in oil, putting in carrots, potatoes, cabbage, celery, Swiss chard, and kale, tomatoes, and seasoning for about twenty minutes.

6. Put in the pureed bean and cook for forty minutes before you put in the rest of the mixture.

7. Put in toasted bread slices. Heat the soup for about twenty minutes.

8. Serve with Parmesan cheese and olive oil.

Nutritional Info: Calories: 418 kcal , Carbohydrates: 41.8 g , Fat: 22 g , Protein: 14 g

56. RICH ONION AND BEEF STEW

Time To Prepare: five minutes

Time to Cook: 10 hours **Yield:** Servings 6

Ingredients:

- 1 beef stock cube

- 1 teaspoon dried mixed herbs (such as Italian seasoning)

- 2 onions, roughly chopped

- 2 pounds (907 g) boneless stewing beef, cut into cubes

- 3 cups water

- 3 tablespoons olive oil, divided • 5 garlic cloves, crushed

- From the cupboard:

- Salt and freshly ground black pepper, to taste

Directions:

1. Grease the insert of the slow cooker with 2 tablespoons of olive oil. Coat a nonstick frying pan with the rest of the olive oil.

2. Heat the oil in the frying pan on moderate to high heat, then put the beef in the frying pan and sear for a couple of minutes or until medium-rare. Shake the frying pan continuously to sear the beef cubes uniformly.

3. Position the cooked beef in the slow cooker, then put in the stock cube, mixed herbs, garlic, onions, salt, black pepper, and water. Stir to mix thoroughly.

4. Place the slow cooker lid on and cook on LOW for ten hours.

5. Ladle the stew in a big container and serve warm.

Nutritional Info: calories: 199 , total fat: 6.3g , carbs: 1.9g , protein: 33.8g

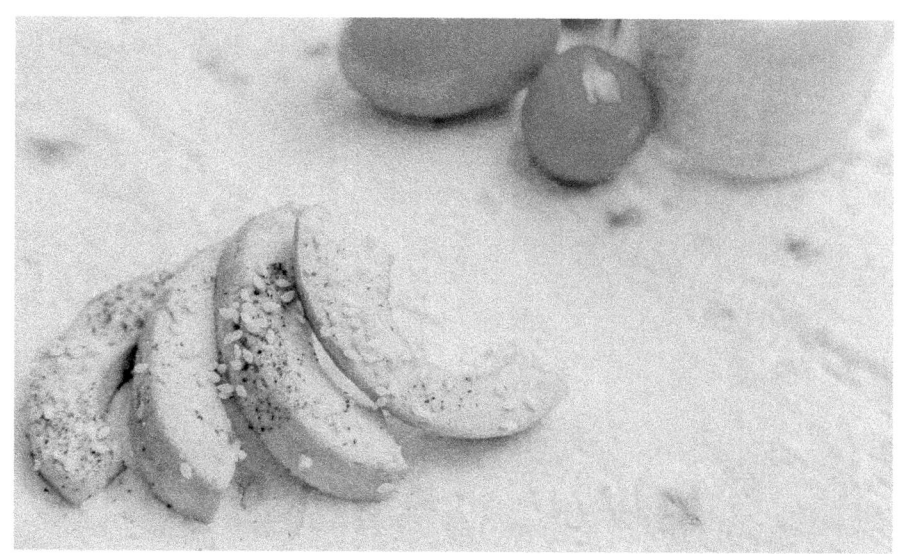

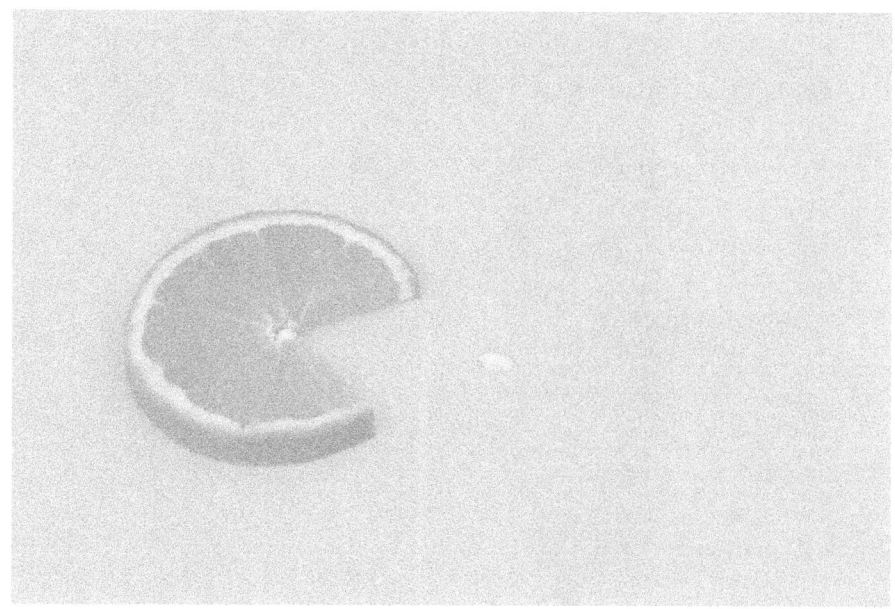

57. ROASTED BUTTERNUT SQUASH APPLE SOUP

Time To Prepare: ten minutes

Time to Cook: forty minutes

Yield: Servings 4

Ingredients:

- 1 butternut squash

- 1 celery rib

- 1 cup water

- 1 small onion

- 1/4 teaspoon cinnamon

- 1/4 teaspoon ginger

- 1/4 teaspoon nutmeg

- 2 red, sweet apples

- 3 cups low-sodium chicken/vegetable stock

- 4 tablespoons olive oil

- Salt & pepper to taste

Directions:

1. Preheat your oven to 400°F.

2. Put diced apple on a one-sheet pan & put the diced butternut squash on the second sheet pan.

3. Allow season to squash olive oil & put in pepper & salt. Stir get everything mix thoroughly. Put in apple with one tablespoon olive oil & stir to coat.

4. Apple & Roast squash for around half an hour, until browned.

5. Heat olive oil (remaining 1 ½ tablespoons) in a big stockpot.

6. Sauté celery & onion for around seven minutes, until soft. Put in Pepper & salt to taste.

7. Put in vegetable or chicken stock & water & bring to a simmer.

8. Once the apple & squash are roasted, put in them to the pot. Put in cinnamon, nutmeg & ginger.

9. Now blend the soup until the desired smoothness is achieved. Season pepper & salt to taste.

10. Serve with desired toppings.

Nutritional Info: Calories: 251 kcal , Protein: 4.06 g , Fat: 15.93 g , Carbohydrates: 25.14 g

58. RUSSIAN CABBAGE SOUP (SHCHI)

Time To Prepare: ten minutes **Time to Cook:** twenty minutes **Yield:** Servings 6

Ingredients:

- ½ big head cabbage, shredded

- ½ teaspoon salt

- 1 (14 oz.) can diced tomatoes with its juice

- 1 bay leaf

- 1 big potato, peeled and diced

- 1 celery stalk, diced

- 1 medium white onion, diced

- 1 tablespoon ghee

- 2 carrots, shredded

- 3 garlic cloves, minced

- 6 cups vegetable broth • Freshly ground black pepper

Directions:

1.   In a huge soup pot using high heat, mix the broth, bay leaf, and potato, and bring to its boiling point.

Lower the heat to low and simmer for fifteen minutes.

2. In the meantime, in a moderate-sized deep cooking pan on moderate heat, heat the ghee. Place the onion and garlic, and sauté for five minutes.

3. Put in the carrots, celery, and cabbage, and cook for a couple of minutes, stirring frequently. Move to the soup pot.

4. Mix in the tomatoes and salt, and flavor with pepper. Mix thoroughly and carry on simmering until all ingredients have become tender and cooked, approximately five minutes. Take off and discard the bay leaf, and serve instantly.

Nutritional Info: Calories: 180 , Total Fat: 3g , Saturated Fat: 2g , Cholesterol: 7mg , Carbohydrates: 20g , Fiber: 5g , Protein: 12g

59. SAFFRON AND SALMON SOUP

Time To Prepare: ten minutes **Time to Cook:** twenty minutes **Yield:** Servings 4

Ingredients:

- ¼ cup extra-virgin olive oil

- ¼ tsp. freshly ground black pepper

- ¼ tsp. saffron threads

- ½ cup dry white wine

- 1 lb. salmon fillets, cut into 1-inch pieces

- 1 tsp. salt

- 2 cups baby spinach

- 2 garlic cloves, thinly cut

- 2 leeks, white parts only, thinly cut

- 2 medium carrots, thinly cut

- 2 tablespoons chopped scallions, both white and green parts

- 2 tablespoons finely chopped fresh flat-leaf parsley

- 4 cups vegetable broth

Directions:

1. In a large pot, heat the oil using high heat.

2. Put in the leeks, carrots, and garlic and sauté until tender, five to seven minutes.

3. Pour the broth then bring to its boiling point.

4. Reduce the heat to a simmer then put in the salmon, salt, pepper, and saffron. Cook until the salmon is thoroughly cooked, minimum 8 minutes.

5. Put in the spinach, wine, scallions, and parsley and cook until the spinach has wilted, one to two minutes, before you serve.

Nutritional Info: Calories: 418 , Total Fat: 26g , Total Carbohydrates: 13g , Sugar: 4g , Fiber: 2g , Protein: 29g , Sodium: 1455mg

60. SLOW COOKER LAMB & CAULIFLOWER SOUP

Time To Prepare: ten minutes

Time to Cook: 4 hours **Yield:** Servings 6

Ingredients:

- ½ teaspoon cracked black pepper

- ½ teaspoon salt 1 cauliflower head, cut into florets

- 1 cup heavy cream

- 1 pound ground lamb

- 1 tablespoon freshly chopped thyme

- 1 yellow onion, chopped

- 2 cloves garlic, chopped 5 cups beef broth

Directions:

1. Put in the ground lamb and cauliflower to the base of a stockpot.

2. Put in in the rest of the ingredients minus the heavy cream, and cook on high for 4 hours.

3. Warm the heavy cream before you put in to the soup. Use an immersion blender to combine the soup until creamy.

Nutritional Info: Calories: 263 , Carbohydrates: 6g , Fiber: 2g Net , Carbohydrates: 4g , Fat: 14g , Protein: 27g

61. SPICY ASIAN-STYLE SOUP

Time To Prepare: ten minutes **Yield:** Servings 4

Ingredients:

½ cup soy milk

½ pound asparagus, diced

1 bay leaf

1 cup celery, diced

1 shallot, diced

1 tablespoon coconut aminos

1 teaspoon Taco seasoning

1/4 teaspoon freshly ground black pepper

- 2 chicken bouillon cubes

- 2 cloves garlic, diced

- 2 cups Crimini mushrooms

- 2 tablespoons butter, softened

- 4 cups water

- Sea salt and black pepper, to taste

Directions:

1. Push the "Sauté" button to heat up your Instant Pot. Once hot, melt the butter; then, sweat the shallot until tender.

2. Mix in garlic; cook an additional 40 seconds, stirring regularly.

3. Put in the rest of the ingredients.

4. Secure the lid. Choose "Manual" mode and High pressure; cook for seven minutes. Once cooking is complete, use a quick pressure release; cautiously remove the lid.

5. Ladle into separate bowls and serve warm. Enjoy!

Nutritional Info: 104 Calories , 7g Fat , 6.6g Total Carbs , 3.9g Protein , 3.5g Sugars

62. SPICY CABBAGE TURMERIC COCONUT SOUP

Time To Prepare: ten minutes **Time to Cook:** twenty minutes **Yield:** Servings 4

Ingredients:

- ½ black pepper ½ teaspoon salt

- 1 head white cabbage

- teaspoon cumin powder

- 1/4 cup coconut milk

- cloves garlic 2 tablespoons coconut oil

- 2 teaspoons turmeric powder • 3 cups vegetable/chicken stock

Directions:

1. Heat the oil in a frying pan on moderate heat.

2. Put in the cabbage & garlic & sauté until the cabbage is delicate.

3. Put in the stock, bubble, spread, & stew for about twenty minutes.

4. Turn off the heat, including the coconut milk & flavors.

5. Blend until the desired smoothness is achieved & season to taste. Serve, gulp & appreciate!

Nutritional Info: Calories: 207 kcal , Protein: 13.52 g , Fat: 10.79 g , Carbohydrates: 16.84 g

63. SPICY LIME-CHICKEN "TORTILLA-LESS" SOUP

Time To Prepare: ten minutes **Time to Cook:** twenty minutes **Yield:** Servings 6

Ingredients:

- ¼ teaspoon cayenne pepper

- ½ teaspoon salt

- 1 (14 oz.) can diced tomatoes, and it's juice

- 1 (4oz.) can diced green chiles

- 1 avocado, cut

- 1 jalapeño pepper, seeded and minced

- 1 m dium white onion, diced

- 1 pound shredded cooked chicken

- 1 tablespoon avocado oil

- 1 teaspoon chili powder

- 1 teaspoon ground cumin

- 3 garlic cloves, minced

- 3 tablespoons freshly squeezed lime juice

- 6 cups chicken broth or vegetable broth

- Fresh cilantro, for decoration

- Freshly ground black pepper

Directions:

1. In a huge soup pot on moderate heat, heat the avocado oil.

2. Put in the garlic, onion, and jalapeño pepper, and sauté for five minutes.

3. Mix in the broth, chicken, tomatoes, green chiles, lime juice, chili powder, cumin, salt, and cayenne pepper, and flavor with black pepper. Put it to a simmer, and cook for about ten minutes.

4. Serve hot, topped with slices of avocado and decorated with cilantro.

Nutritional Info: Calories: 283 , Total Fat: 7g , Saturated Fat: 1g , Cholesterol: 47mg , Carbohydrates: 12g , Fiber: 3g , Protein: 29g

64. SPICY RAMEN NOODLES

Time To Prepare: fifteen minutes

Time to Cook: 0 minutes **Yield:** Servings 4

Ingredients:

- • ¼ cup chopped fresh cilantro

- ¼ cup cut scallion

- ¼ cup thinly cut cucumber

- 1 tablespoon coconut aminos

- 1 tablespoon freshly squeezed lime juice

- 1 tablespoon grated peeled fresh ginger

- 1 tablespoon raw honey

- chili powder

- tablespoons rice vinegar

- 2 tablespoons sesame oil

- 2 tablespoons sesame seeds

- 8 ounces buckwheat noodles or rice noodles, cooked

Directions:

1. In a big serving container, meticulously mix the noodles, sesame seeds, cucumber, scallion, cilantro, sesame oil, vinegar, ginger, coconut aminos, honey, lime juice, and chili powder.

2. Split among 4 soup bowls and serve at room temperature.

Nutritional Info: Calories: 663 , Total Fat: 28g , Saturated Fat: 4g , Cholesterol: 0mg , Carbohydrates: 115g , Fiber: 39g , Protein: 21g

65. SPICY SEAFOOD STEW

Time To Prepare: ten minutes **Time to Cook:** twenty minutes **Yield:** Servings 6

Ingredients:

- ¼ cup freshly squeezed lime juice

- ½ cup chopped fresh cilantro

- ½ cup chopped yellow onion

- ½ cup coconut milk

- ½ cup diced green pepper

- ½ cup thinly cut scallions

- ¾ pound medium-size shrimp, shelled and deveined

- ¾ pound skinless firm-fleshed fish fillets, (cod, center-cut salmon, or halibut)

- 1 tablespoon minced garlic

- teaspoon hot pepper sauce tablespoons olive oil

- cups canned peeled, chopped tomatoes, undrained

- Seasoned salt, to taste

Directions:

1.   Warm the oil in a huge nonstick frying pan on moderate to high heat. Put in the onions, green pepper, garlic, and tomatoes. Put to a

simmer while stirring once in a while, then cook for three to four minutes.

2.   Put in the coconut milk, pepper sauce, lime juice, and seasoned salt. Set to a simmer and cook for minimum 2 minutes. Put in the fish and stir, being cautious not to break apart the fillets. Cook till the fish is thoroughly cooked, approximately eight minutes. Put in the shrimp and cook until opaque and thoroughly cooked, approximately five minutes.

3.   To serve, use a slotted spoon to take equal amounts of the fish and shrimp to 4 shallow serving bowls. Place the sauce over the seafood and decorate with scallions and cilantro. Serve hot.

Nutritional Info: Calories: 219 , Fat: 11 g , Protein: 19g , Sodium: 375 mg , Fiber: 2 g , Carbohydrates: 10 g

66. SWEET POTATO AND BLACK BEAN CHILI

Time To Prepare: ten minutes **Time to Cook:** twenty minutes **Yield:** Servings 8

Ingredients:

- ¼ teaspoon cayenne pepper

- ¼ teaspoon dried oregano

- ½ teaspoon ground cinnamon

- 1 (28-ounce) can diced tomatoes with their juice

- 1 green bell pepper, diced

- 1 red bell pepper, diced

- 1 red onion, diced

- 1 tablespoon chili powder

- 1 tablespoon freshly squeezed lime juice

- 1 e   cocoa powder

- 1 teaspoon ground cumin

- 1 teaspoon salt

- 2 cups vegetable broth

- 2 tablespoons avocado oil

- 3 cups black beans, drained and washed well

- 3 cups cooked sweet potato cubes

- 5 garlic cloves, minced

Directions:

1. In a huge soup pot on moderate heat, warm the avocado oil.

2. Place the onion and garlic, and sauté for a couple of minutes.

3. Mix in the red bell pepper and the green bell pepper, and sauté for approximately 3 minutes until tender.

4. Put in the sweet potato, beans, broth, tomatoes, lime juice, chili powder, cocoa powder, cumin, salt, cinnamon, cayenne pepper, and oregano, then stir until blended. Put to a simmer, and cook for fifteen minutes. Serve instantly.

Nutritional Info: Calories: 160 , Total Fat: 4g , Saturated Fat: 0g , Cholesterol: 0mg , Carbohydrates: 29g , Fiber: 6g , Protein: 8g

67.   SWEET POTATO AND CORN SOUP

Time To Prepare: ten minutes **Time to Cook:** twenty minutes **Yield:** Servings 4

Ingredients:

- ¼ cup extra-virgin olive oil or coconut oil

- ¼ teaspoon freshly ground black pepper

- 1 cup broccoli florets

- 1 cup coconut milk or almond milk

- 1 cup frozen corn kernels

- 1 cup thinly cut mushrooms

- 1 medium zucchini, cut into ¼-inch dice

- 1 small onion, cut into ¼-inch dice

- 1 teaspoon salt

- 2 cups peeled sweet potatoes cut into ¼-inch dice

- 2 tablespoons finely chopped fresh flat-leaf parsley

- 4 cups vegetable broth

Directions:

1. In a large pot, heat the oil on high heat.

2. Put in the zucchini, broccoli, mushrooms, and onion and sauté until tender, 5 to 8 minutes.

3. Pour the broth and sweet potatoes and place it to its boiling point.

4. Lower the heat to a simmer and cook until the sweet potatoes are soft, five to seven minutes.

5. Put in the corn, coconut milk, parsley, salt, and pepper. Cook on low heat up to the corn is thoroughly heated before you serve.

Nutritional Info: Calories: 402 , Total Fat: 29g , Total Carbohydrates: 31g , Sugar: 9g , Fiber: 6g , Protein: 10g , Sodium: 1406mg

68.   TEX-MEX CHICKEN SOUP

Time To Prepare: ten minutes

Time to Cook: 1 hour **Yield:** Servings 4

Ingredients:

- ¼ cup roasted pumpkin seeds

- 1 teaspoon paprika powder

- 1 yellow onion, chopped

- 1¾ cups coconut cream

- 12 ounces (340 g) boneless chicken thighs

- tablespoons coconut oil

- tablespoons Tex-Mex seasoning

- tablespoons lime juice

- Fresh cilantro, chopped Salt nd ground black pepper, to taste

Directions:

1.   Cook the chicken thighs in a pot of water, covered, for thirty minutes or until the chicken is completely fork-soft. Move the chicken to a container and reserve the chicken broth until ready to use.

2.   Warm the coconut oil in a nonstick frying pan on moderate heat, then put in the onion and drizzle with Tex-Mex seasoning, salt, and pepper. sauté for five minutes until the onion is translucent.

3.   Pour over the reserved chicken broth and coconut cream. Bring them to a simmer for about twenty minutes or until it becomes thick.

4.   Put in the chicken, pumpkin seeds, paprika powder, lime juice, and cilantro to the soup. Stir to blend well before you serve.

Nutritional Info: calories: 730 , total fat: 63g , net carbs: 19g , fiber: 9g , protein: 23g

69.   THAI CHICKEN NOODLE SOUP

Time To Prepare: ten minutes

Time to Cook: ten minutes **Yield:** Servings 2-3

Ingredients:

- 6 cups low-sodium chicken broth

- 1 stalk lemongrass, minced

- 1 bay leaf

- 1 tablespoon ginger, grated

- 1 big carrot, cut

- 1 cup broccoli florets, trimmed

- 1 cup mushrooms, quartered

- ½ teaspoon. cayenne pepper

- 3 cloves garlic, minced

- 2 Tablespoon. gluten-free soy sauce Salt and black pepper (to taste) a handful of fresh cilantro, chopped 1-2 fresh chicken breasts, chopped

- 1/4 cup fresh lime juice

- 1/4 cup coconut milk 8-10 oz. gluten-free flat Thai rice noodles

Directions:

1.   Boil noodles in accordance with package directions, or until firm to the bite. Drain and save for later.

2. Pour chicken broth in a big pot and bring to its boiling point using high heat. Put in chicken, broccoli, mushrooms, lemongrass, ginger, carrot, bay leaf. Turn heat to high and let the broth boil for a minute. Cover the pot and decrease the heat to moderate. Simmer the soup for 6 more minutes.

3. While the soup is simmering, mix in cayenne, garlic, lime juice, and soy sauce. Turn heat to low and put in the coconut milk; stir thoroughly.

4. Put cooked noodles into bowls. Pour soup over the noodles, then drizzle with cilantro.

Nutritional Info: Calories: 503 kcal , Protein: 48.11 g , Fat: 19.63 g , Carbohydrates: 35.9 g

70. THAI WINTER VEGETABLE SOUP

Time To Prepare: 60 minutes

Time to Cook: 6 hours **Yield:** Servings 12

Ingredients:

- • ½ Of Lemon Juice

- 1 Lime Juice

- 1 Piece Ginger (Peeled, Grated)

- 1 Teaspoon Cumin

- 14 Ounce Coconut Milk

- 14 Ounce Peeled Italian Plum Tomatoes

- 2 Large Onions (Peeled, Quartered)

- 2 St lks Lemongrass (Split)

- 3 Carrots (Peeled, Chopped)

- 3 Cloves Garlic (Peeled, Chopped)

- 3 Red Bell Peppers (Quartered, Seeded)

- 4 Large Sweet Potatoes (Peeled, Cut)

- 4 Tablespoons Cilantro (Chopped)

- Ground Black Pepper

- Optional: 1 Green Chili Pepper (Chopped)

- Salt

Directions:

1. Cook the vegetables with ginger and chili before pouring in coconut milk.

2. Mix in cilantro, cumin, lemon juice, and seasoning, cooking for around six hours.

3. Remove lemongrass and blend until thick.

4. Put in lime juice, seasoning, and cilantro to serve.

Nutritional Info: Calories: 468 kcal , Carbohydrates: 81 g , Fat: fifteen g , Protein: 8.5 g

71. TOMATO AND BASIL SOUP

Time To Prepare: five minutes

Time to Cook: fifteen minutes **Yield:** Servings 4

- ¼ cup chopped fresh basil leaves

- ¼ cup heavy whipping cream

- 1 (14.5-ounce / 411-g) can diced tomatoes

- 2 ounces (57 g) cream cheese • 4 tablespoons butter

- From the cupboard:

- Salt and freshly ground black pepper, to taste

Directions:

1. Position the diced tomatoes in a food processor. Process until the desired smoothness is achieved.

2. Melt the butter in a deep cooking pan on moderate heat. Put in the tomato purée, cream, and cheese. Cook for about ten minutes or until well blended. Keep stirring during the cooking.

3. Drizzle with chopped basil leaves, salt, and black pepper. Keep cooking for another five minutes or until the desired smoothness is achieved and the soup has become thick. Stir continuously.

4. Ladle the soup into a big container and serve warm.

Nutritional Info: calories: 238 , total fat: 22.1g , total carbs: 8.9g , fiber: 2.1g , net carbs: 6.8g , protein: 3.1g

72.   TOMATO BISQUE SOUP

Time To Prepare: ten minutes

Time to Cook: forty minutes **Yield:** Servings 6

Ingredients:

- 1 cup heavy cream

- 1 teaspoon freshly chopped thyme

- 2 tablespoons butter

- 3 cloves garlic, chopped

- 3 cups canned whole, peeled tomatoes

- 4 cups chicken broth • Salt & black pepper, to taste

Directions:

1. Put in the butter to the bottom of a stockpot.

2. Put in in all the rest of the ingredients minus the heavy cream. Bring to its boiling point, and then simmer for forty minutes.

3. Warm the heavy cream, and then mix into the soup.

Nutritional Info: Calories: 144 , Carbohydrates: 4g , Fiber: 1g Net , Carbohydrates: 3g , Fat: 12g , Protein: 4g

73.   TURKEY MEATBALL SOUP

Time To Prepare: fifteen minutes

Time to Cook: fifteen minutes **Yield:** Servings 6

For the Meatballs:

- ¼ teaspoon red pepper flakes

- ½ teaspoon dried oregano

- ½ teaspoon salt

- 1 pound ground turkey

- 1 tablespoon Dijon mustard

- 1 tablespoon ghee

- 1 teaspoon dried basil

- 1 teaspoon garlic powder • Freshly ground black pepper

For the Soup:

- ½ teaspoon dried thyme

- 1 bay leaf

- 1 medium white onion, diced

- 2 carrots, diced

- 2 cups shredded kale leaves, stemmed and meticulously washed

- 2 garlic cloves, minced

- 6 cups vegetable broth **Directions:**

To make the Meatballs:

1. In a moderate-sized container, put the turkey, mustard, basil, garlic powder, oregano, salt, and red pepper flakes, and flavor with pepper. With your hands, combine the ingredients until they are well blended.

2. Put in the ghee to a stockpot on moderate to high heat. Roll the meat mixture into 1-inch balls and layer across the bottom of the pot. Cook for minimum 2 minutes per side, until almost thoroughly cooked. Move the meatballs to a plate.

To make the Soup:

1. To the stockpot, put in the onion, carrots, garlic, and thyme. Cook for approximately 2 minutes, slowly stirring, until the onions are translucent.

2. Put in the broth, kale, bay leaf, and meatballs. Put to a simmer, lessen the heat to moderate-low and simmer for approximately fifteen minutes until the meatballs are thoroughly cooked, and the kale has tenderized. Remove and discard the bay leaf. Serve hot.

Nutritional Info: Calories: 259 , Total Fat: 14g , Saturated Fat: 5g , Cholesterol: 88mg , Carbohydrates: 9g , Fiber: 2g , Protein: 26g

74.   TUSCAN STYLE SOUP

Time To Prepare: three minutes

Time to Cook: five minutes **Yield:** Servings 4

Ingredients:

- ½ cup leeks, cut

- 1 carrot, trimmed and grated

- 1 zucchini, shredded

- 1/4 teaspoon ground black pepper

- 2 cups broth, if possible homemade

- 2 cups water

- 2 garlic cloves, minced

- 2 tablespoons butter, melted

- 4 cups broccoli rabe, broken into pieces

- Sea salt, to taste

Directions:

1. Push the "Sauté" button to heat up your Instant Pot; now, melt the butter.

Cook the leeks for approximately 2 minutes or until tender.

2. Put in minced garlic and cook an additional 40 seconds.

3. Put in the rest of the ingredients. Secure the lid.

4. "Manual" mode and Low pressure; cook for about three minutes. Once cooking is complete, use a quick pressure release; cautiously remove the lid. Enjoy!

Nutritional Info: 95 Calories , 6.7g Fat , 5.2g Total Carbs , 4.2g Protein , 1.4g Sugars

75. VEGETABLE BEEF SOUP

Time To Prepare: ten minutes

Time to Cook: 4-6 hours **Yield:** Servings 6

Ingredients:

- ½ cup diced tomatoes

- 1 pound lean ground beef

- 1 teaspoon freshly chopped rosemary

- 1 teaspoon freshly chopped thyme

- 1 yellow onion, chopped

- 1 zucchini, diced

- 2 cloves garlic, chopped

- 2 stalks celery, chopped

- 4 cups beef broth • Salt & pepper, to taste

Directions:

1. Put in all the ingredients to a slow cooker and cook on high for four to 6 hours.

2. Stir thoroughly before you serve.

Nutritional Info: Calories: 185 , Carbohydrates: 5g , Fiber: 1g Net , Carbohydrates: 4g , Fat: 6g , Protein: 7g

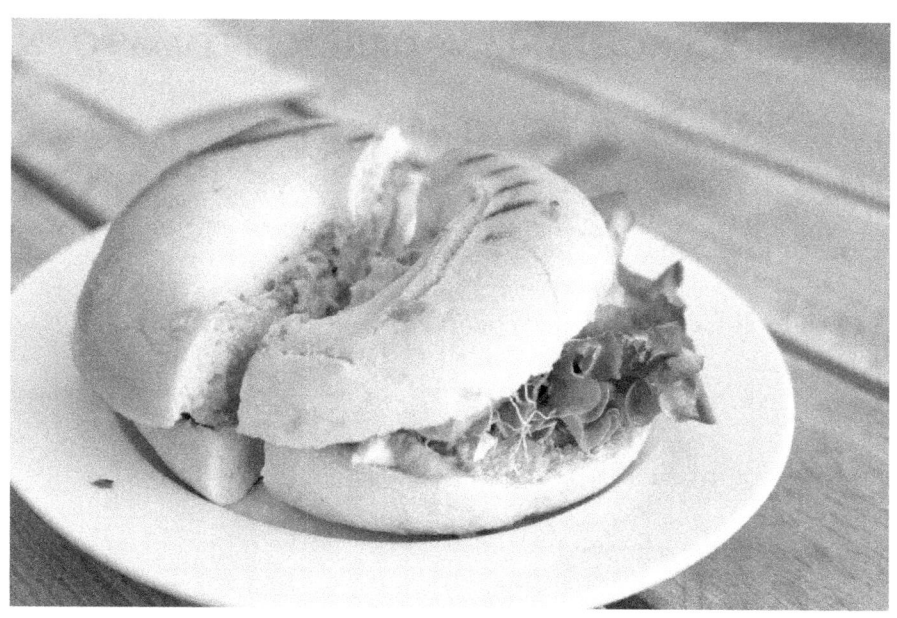

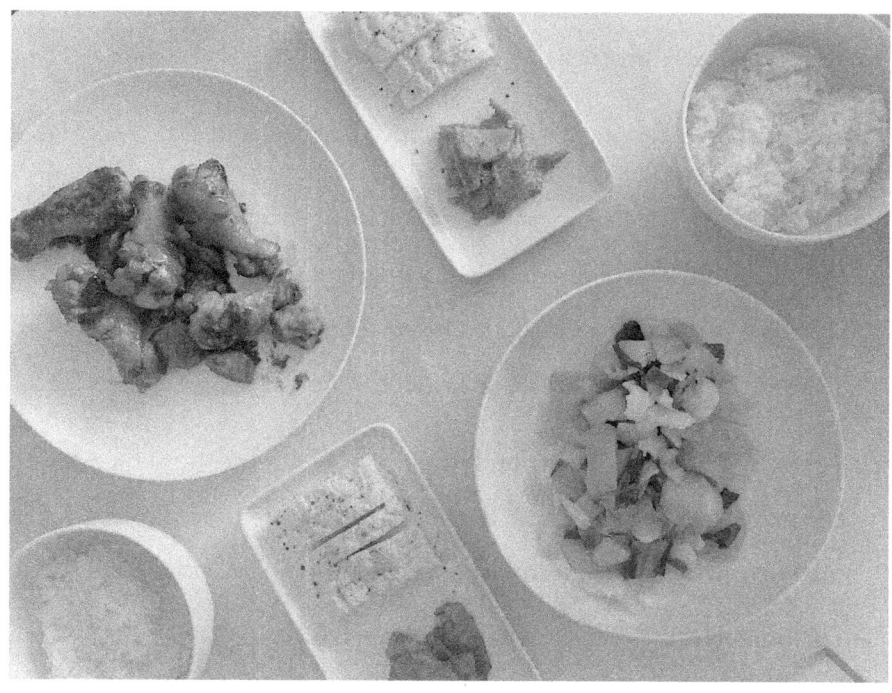

76. VEGETARIAN GARLIC, TOMATO & ONION SOUP

Time To Prepare: fifteen minutes

Time to Cook: thirty minutes **Yield:** Servings 6

- ½ cup full-fat unsweetened coconut milk

- 1 bay leaf

- 1 teaspoon Italian seasoning

- 1 yellow onion, chopped

- 1½ cups canned diced tomatoes

- 3 cloves garlic, chopped

- 6 cups vegetable broth

- Fresh basil, for serving • Pinch of salt & pepper, to taste

Directions:

1. Put in all the ingredients minus the coconut milk and fresh basil to a stockpot on moderate heat and bring to its boiling point. Reduce to a simmer and cook for half an hour

2. Take away the bay leaf, and then use an immersion blender to combine the soup until the desired smoothness is achieved. Mix in the coconut milk.Decorate using fresh basil before you serve.

Nutritional Info: Calories: 104 , Carbohydrates: 6g , Fiber: 1g Net , Carbohydrates: 5g , Fat: 7g , Protein: 6g

77.   WEDDING SOUP

Time To Prepare: fifteen minutes

Time to Cook: 60 minutes **Yield:** Servings 6

Ingredients:

- ¼ bunch fresh parsley, chopped

- ¾ pound lean ground beef

- 1 cup rough chopped fresh spinach with stems removed

- 1 egg or ¼ cup egg substitute

- 1 yellow onion, chopped

- 2 quarts Rich Poultry Stock or low-sodium canned chicken stock

- 2 sprigs fresh basil, chopped

- 3 cloves garlic, minced

- 3 slices Italian bread, toasted

- 3 sprigs fresh oregano, chopped

- 4 ounces fresh grated Parmesan cheese

- Freshly cracked black pepper, to taste

Directions:

1. Preheat your oven to 375°F.

2. Wet the toasted Italian bread with water, then squeeze out all the liquid. 3. In a big container, combine the bread, beef, egg, onion,

garlic, parsley, oregano, basil, pepper, and half of the Parmesan. Form the mixture into 1- to two-inch balls; put in a baking dish and cook for twenty minutes to half an hour. Take off from the oven and drain using paper towels.

4. Steam the spinach firm to the bite. In a big stockpot, mix the stock, spinach, and meatballs; simmer for half an hour

5. Ladle the soup into serving bowls then top with the rest of the cheese

Nutritional Info: Calories: 245 , Fat: 10 g , Protein: 26 g , Sodium: 1,021 mg , Fiber: 0.5 g , Carbohydrates: 9 g

78.   WHITE VELVET CAULIFLOWER SOUP

Time To Prepare: ten minutes **Time to Cook:** twenty minutes **Yield:** Servings 6

Ingredients:

• 1 head cauliflower, chopped into 1-inch pieces

  1 small celery root, peeled, cut into 1-inch pieces

  1 small white onion, diced

  1 tbsp. avocado oil

  2 scallions, cut

  2 tbsp. ghee

• 3 garlic cloves, minced

• 4 cups vegetable broth

Directions:

1. In a huge soup pot on moderate heat, heat the avocado oil.

2. Place the onion and garlic, and sauté for five minutes.

3. Place the celery root and cauliflower.

4. Raise the heat to moderate-high, then continue to sauté for minimum five minutes, or until the cauliflower starts to brown and caramelize the sides.

5. Mix in the broth and ghee and place it to its boiling point. Lessen the heat to moderate-low and simmer for about ten minutes. Take away the pot from the heat.

6. Use an immersion blender to or in batches in a standard blender, purée the soup until creamy. Serve instantly, sprinkled with the scallions.

Nutritional Info: Calories: 183 , Total Fat: 8g , Saturated Fat: 3g , Cholesterol: 0mg , Carbohydrates: 10g , Fiber: 3g , Protein: 9g

79. WHOLESOME CABBAGE SOUP

Time To Prepare: two minutes

Time to Cook: 8 minutes **Yield:** Servings 4

Ingredients:

- ½ pound Capocollo, chopped

- ½ teaspoon cayenne pepper

- 1 bay leaf

- 1 celery stalk, chopped

- 1 cup tomatoes, puréed

- 1 cup water

  1 onion, chopped

  1 parsnip, chopped

  1 pound cabbage, cut into wedges

  2 cups broth, if possible homemade

  Coarse sea salt and ground black pepper, to your preference

Directions:

1. Put in all of the above ingredients to your Instant Pot.

2. Secure the lid. Choose "Manual" mode and High pressure; cook for about three minutes. Once cooking is complete, use a quick pressure release; cautiously remove the lid.

3. Ladle into four soup bowls and serve hot. Enjoy!

Nutritional Info: 258 Calories , 20.4g Fat , 6g Total Carbs , 9.9g Protein , 3.6g Sugars

80.   ZESTY BROCCOLI SOUP

Time To Prepare: ten minutes **Time to Cook:** twenty minutes **Yield:** Servings 4

Ingredients:

- ½ teaspoon freshly squeezed lemon juice

- ½ teaspoon lemon zest

- ½ teaspoon salt

- 1 carrot, chopped

- 1 celery stalk, diced

- 1 head broccoli, roughly chopped

- 1 medium white onion, diced

- 1 tablespoon ghee

- 3 cups vegetable broth

- 3 garlic cloves, minced • Freshly ground black pepper

Directions:

1. In a huge soup pot on moderate heat, melt the ghee.

2. Place the onion and garlic, and sauté for five minutes.

3. Put in the broccoli, carrot, and celery, and sauté for a couple of minutes.

4. Mix in the broth, salt, lemon juice, and lemon zest, and flavor with pepper. Heat to a simmer, and cook for minimum ten minutes. Serve instantly.

Nutritional Info: Calories: 80 , Total Fat: 4g , Saturated Fat: 2g , Cholesterol: 0mg , Carbohydrates: 10g , Fiber: 3g , Protein: 2g

81.   STRAWBERRY SOUFFLÉ

Time To Prepare: fifteen minutes

Time to Cook: twelve minutes **Yield:** Servings 6

Ingredients:

- 18 ounces of fresh strawberries, hulled

- 5 organic egg whites, divided

- 4 teaspoons of fresh lemon juice

- 1/3 cup of raw honey, divided

Directions:

1. Preheat your oven to 350F.

2. Place the strawberries in a blender then pulse until a puree form.

3. Strain the strawberry puree using a strainer while discarding the seeds.

4. Mix the strawberry puree to three tablespoons of honey, two egg whites, and fresh lemon juice. Pulse until a frothy and light-weight develops.

5. Beat the eggs in a separate container up to it becomes frothy.

6. Put in the remaining honey and beat until a stiff peak forms.

7. Gently- fold the egg whites into the strawberry mixture.

8. Move the mixture toto six big ramekins and place them on a baking sheet.

9. Bake for around 10-twelve minutes.

10. Take out of the oven and serve instantly.

Nutritional Info: , Calories: 100 , Fat: 0.3g , Carbohydrates: 22.3g , Sugar: 19.9g , Protein: 3.7g , Sodium: 30mg

CPSIA information can be obtained
at www.ICGtesting.com
Printed in the USA
BVHW041515190321
602997BV00010B/534